INTRODUCTORY ENDOCRINOLOGY
A Concise and Applied Digest

INTRODUCTORY ENDOCRINOLOGY
A Concise and Applied Digest

Authors

Romesh Khardori MD PhD FACP FRCP(C)

Professor of Medicine
Division of Endocrinology and Metabolism
Department of Internal Medicine
Eastern Virginia Medical School
Norfolk, Virginia, United States

DD Bansal MSc PhD

Former Professor and Head
Department of Biochemistry
Panjab University and
Government Medical College and Hospital
Chandigarh, India

Pranav Mehra MSc PhD

Guest Faculty
Department of Biochemistry
Panjab University
Chandigarh, India

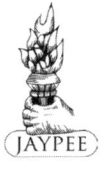

The Health Sciences Publisher
New Delhi | London | Panama

Jaypee Brothers Medical Publishers (P) Ltd

Headquarters

Jaypee Brothers Medical Publishers (P) Ltd
4838/24, Ansari Road, Daryaganj
New Delhi 110 002, India
Phone: +91-11-43574357
Fax: +91-11-43574314
Email: jaypee@jaypeebrothers.com

Overseas Offices

J.P. Medical Ltd
83 Victoria Street, London
SW1H 0HW (UK)
Phone: +44 20 3170 8910
Fax: +44 (0)20 3008 6180
Email: info@jpmedpub.com

Jaypee-Highlights Medical Publishers Inc
City of Knowledge, Bld. 237, Clayton
Panama City, Panama
Phone: +1 507-301-0496
Fax: +1 507-301-0499
Email: cservice@jphmedical.com

Jaypee Brothers Medical Publishers (P) Ltd
17/1-B Babar Road, Block-B, Shaymali
Mohammadpur, Dhaka-1207
Bangladesh
Mobile: +08801912003485
Email: jaypeedhaka@gmail.com

Jaypee Brothers Medical Publishers (P) Ltd
Bhotahity, Kathmandu
Nepal
Phone: +977-9741283608
Email: kathmandu@jaypeebrothers.com

Website: www.jaypeebrothers.com
Website: www.jaypeedigital.com

© 2018, Jaypee Brothers Medical Publishers

The views and opinions expressed in this book are solely those of the original contributor(s)/author(s) and do not necessarily represent those of editor(s) of the book.

All rights reserved. No part of this publication and Interactive DVD-ROM may be reproduced, stored or transmitted in any form or by any means, electronic, mechanical, photocopying, recording or otherwise, without the prior permission in writing of the publishers.

All brand names and product names used in this book are trade names, service marks, trademarks or registered trademarks of their respective owners. The publisher is not associated with any product or vendor mentioned in this book.

Medical knowledge and practice change constantly. This book is designed to provide accurate, authoritative information about the subject matter in question. However, readers are advised to check the most current information available on procedures included and check information from the manufacturer of each product to be administered, to verify the recommended dose, formula, method and duration of administration, adverse effects and contraindications. It is the responsibility of the practitioner to take all appropriate safety precautions. Neither the publisher nor the author(s)/editor(s) assume any liability for any injury and/or damage to persons or property arising from or related to use of material in this book.

This book is sold on the understanding that the publisher is not engaged in providing professional medical services. If such advice or services are required, the services of a competent medical professional should be sought.

Every effort has been made where necessary to contact holders of copyright to obtain permission to reproduce copyright material. If any have been inadvertently overlooked, the publisher will be pleased to make the necessary arrangements at the first opportunity. The **CD/DVD-ROM** (if any) provided in the sealed envelope with this book is complimentary and free of cost. **Not meant for sale**.

Inquiries for bulk sales may be solicited at: jaypee@jaypeebrothers.com

Introductory Endocrinology: *A Concise and Applied Digest* / Romesh Khardori, DD Bansal, Pranav Mehra

First Edition: **2018**

ISBN: 978-93-5270-094-3

Printed at Rajkamal Electric Press, Plot No. 2, Phase-IV, Kundli, Haryana.

Dedicated to

*Studen/ts/Learners
In Pursuit of Knowledge*

Preface

In the last 5 decades, endocrinology has gained ascendancy primarily due to refinements in our assay techniques, revolutionary shifts in cellular biology, and the genomics. It remains to date one of the most fascinating specialties in biology due to intricacies of feed forward and feedback system that are both challenging and exciting all at once. It is heavily rooted in physiology, cellular biology, and biochemistry. Those who have made endocrinology a subject of their fancy often tell you how rewarding the cerebral study of endocrinology is, both at bench as well as in the clinic/bedside. Study of endocrinology is no longer restricted to traditional endocrine gland, but also brings under its ambit study of transcellular and intercellular communication (cytokines, chemokines, intracellular signal transduction, hormonal control of immunoregulatory systems). Endocrinologists now have tools available by which they can assess signaling systems without having to sacrifice whole animal. This includes dynamic imaging and tissue sampling *in vivo*.

Endocrinology is taught at undergraduate (college bound students), graduate level (medical students, postgraduate, and PhD students in subjects like biochemistry and zoology). Physicians willing to specialize in endocrinology obtain and complete fellowship in endocrinology (2–3 years following completion of MD in medicine or pediatrics). However, many students find study of endocrinology daunting because they are left at the mercy of textbooks that are often too detailed and lack the rhythm of taking student through understanding of basic building blocks. Keeping this in mind, we designed this short book to facilitate transition from novice to beginner at all levels.

This book is a product of a long and long-distance friendship between two of the authors (Drs Bansal and Khardori) who met nearly 4 decades ago while thrown together in the laboratory of Professor JS Bajaj at the All India Institute of Medical Sciences, New Delhi, India. Professor Bajaj's meticulous attention to details was no less instrumental in sparking our interest in endocrinology/biochemistry. This book also takes into account concerns and interactions of a teacher and his graduate student, and the lessons learned in the process (Professor Bansal and Dr Mehra).

We hope the readers will find it simple to read and easy to grasp facilitating their transition as well as strengthening the concepts and appreciation of basic principles that operate to make the system whole.

We welcome any suggestions from the readers to improve the scope and the reach of this book.

Romesh Khardori
DD Bansal
Pranav Mehra

Acknowledgment

Authors are grateful to Mrs Jyoti Mehra, Technical Officer, Multimedia and Animation Department, Centre for Development of Advanced Computing, Mohali for helping in designing the diagrams presented in this book.

Contents

1. Introduction — 1
2. Hormone Receptors — 19
3. Hypothalamus — 33
4. Pituitary Gland — 37
5. Thyroid Gland — 50
6. Adrenal Gland — 62
7. Hormones Regulating Calcium Metabolism — 76
8. Pancreas — 87
9. Gonads — 104
10. Adipose Tissue Hormones — 117
11. Pineal Gland — 123
12. Gastrointestinal Tract Hormones — 125
13. Hormones from Liver — 131
14. Hormones from Kidney — 133
15. Hormones from Heart — 137
16. Vitamin A — 141
17. Prostaglandins — 143

18.	Nitric Oxide	146
19.	Endocrine Tumors	149
20.	Growth Factors	157
	Appendix	*167*
	Index	*169*

Nobel Prizes for Research in Endocrinology

Year	Nobel prize winner	Pioneer work
2012	Robert Lefkowitz	For his studies on G-protein coupled receptors
1998	Robert F Furchgott, Louis J Ignarro, and Ferid Murad	For discovering nitric oxide as a signaling molecule
1994	Alfred G Gilman and Martin Rodbell	For discovering G-proteins and their role in signal transduction
1992	Edmond H Fischer and Edwin G Krebs	For discovering reversible protein phosphorylation as a biological regulatory mechanism
1986	Stanley Cohen and Rita Levi-Montalcini	For discovering growth factors
1982	Sune K Bergström, Bengt I Samuelsson, and John R Vane	For discovering prostaglandins and related biologically active molecules
1977	Rosalyn S Yalow SHARED WITH Roger Guillemin and Andrew V Schally	For development of radioimmunoassay of insulin For discovering peptide hormone production in brain
1971	Earl W Sutherland, Jr.	For discovering mechanism of hormone action
1958	Frederick Sanger	For discovering structure of insulin
1950	Edward C Kendall, Tadeus Reichstein, and Philip S Hench	For discovering hormones of adrenal cortex, their structure, and biological action

Continued

Continued

Year	Nobel prize winner	Pioneer work
1947	Bernardo A Houssay	For discovering role of hormone of anterior pituitary lobe in the metabolism of sugar
1939	Adolf FJ Butenandt	Shared for his research on sex hormones
1923	Frederick G Banting and John JR Macleod	For discovering insulin
1909	Emil T Kocher	For his work on physiology, pathology, and surgery of thyroid gland

Abbreviations

25-OH D3	25-hydroxycholecalciferol
3β-OHSD	3β-hydroxysteroid dehydrogenase
AAA system	Inter-relationship amongst angiotensin, aldosterone, and atrial natriuretic peptide
ACTH	Adrenocorticotropic hormone
ADH	Antidiuretic hormone
ADP	Adenosine diphosphate
AIP	Aryl-hydrocarbon receptor interacting protein gene
AMH	Anti-Müllerian hormone
ANF	Atrial natriuretic factor
ANP	Atrial natriuretic peptide
AP	Alkaline phosphatase
Arg	Arginine
Asp	Aspartate
ATP	Adenosine triphosphate
AVP	Arginine vasopressin
BDNF	Brain-derived neurotrophic factor
BMR	Basal metabolic rate
BNP	Brain natriuretic peptide
cAMP	Cyclic adenosine monophosphate
CaSR	Calcium sensing receptor
CBG	Corticosteroid binding globulin
cGMP	Cyclic guanosine monophosphate
CGRP	Calcitonin gene-related peptide
CMIA	Chemiluminescent microparicle immunoassay
CNP	C-type natriuretic peptide
CNS	Central nervous system
Co-SMAD	Common-mediated SMADs
CREB protein	cAMP responsive element binding protein
CRF	Corticotropin releasing factor

CRH	Corticotropin releasing hormone
DAG	Diacylglycerol
DHT	Dihydrotestosterone
DIT	Di-iodothyronine
DNA	Deoxyribonucleic acid
E1	Estrone
E2	Estradiol
E3	Estriol
EGF	Epidermal growth factor
EGFR	Epidermal growth factor receptor
ELISA	Enzyme-linked immunosorbent assay
ER	Endoplasmic reticulum
ET-1	Endothelin-1
FGF	Fibroblast growth factor
FPIR	First phase of insulin release
FSH	Follicle stimulating hormone
GDP	Guanosine diphosphate
GH	Growth hormone
GHRH	Growth hormone releasing hormone
GIP	Glucose-dependent insulinotropic polypeptide
GIT	Gastrointestinal tract
GLP	Glucagon-like peptide
GLUT2	Glucose transporter 2
GnRH	Gonadotropin releasing hormone
GPCR	G-protein coupled receptor
GRE	Glucocorticoid response element
GTP	Guanosine-5'-triphosphate
HbA1c	Glycosylated hemoglobin
hCG	Human chorionic gonadotropin
HCl	Hydrochloric acid
HGF	Hepatocyte growth factor
hGR	Human glucocorticoid receptor
HIF	Hypoxia inducible factor
HPA	Hypothalamic-pituitary-adrenal
HRE	Hormone response element
HRP	Horseradish peroxidase

HSP	Heat shock protein
IAPP	Islet amyloid polypeptide
IGF	Insulin-like growth factor
IP3	Inositol triphosphate
IRS	Insulin receptor substrate
IVF	*In vitro* fertilization
JAK-2	Janus kinase 2
LH	Luteinizing hormone
LTBP	Latent TGF-β binding protein
MAD	Mothers against decapentaplegic
MCT	Medullary carcinoma thyroid
MEN	Multiple endocrine neoplasia
MIH	Müllerian inhibitory substance
MIT	Monoiodothyronine
MODY	Maturity onset diabetes
mRNA	Messenger RNA
MSH	Melanocyte stimulating hormone
NCoR	Nuclear receptor corepressor
NF1	Neurofibromatosis type 1 gene
NGF	Nerve growth factor
NO	Nitric oxide
NR3	Nuclear subfamily 3
NT	Neurotrophins
OXTR	Oxytocin receptors
PDGF	Platelet-derived growth factor
PDK-1	Phosphoinositide-dependent kinase-1
PG	Prostaglandin
PIP2	Phosphoinositide biphosphate
PKA	Protein kinase A
PKB	Protein kinase B
PL	Phospholipase
PLC	Phospholipase C
PLCγ	Phospholipase Cγ
PLGF	Placental growth factor
PNET	Pancreatic neuroendocrine tumor
PNS	Peripheral nervous system

POMC	Pro-opiomelanocortin
PP	Pancreatic polypeptide
PPNAD	Pigmented nodular adrenocortical disease
PRKARIA	Regulatory subunit 1-α of the protein kinase A
ProANP	Pro-atrial natriuretic peptide
ProPTH	Proparathormone
PTH	Parathyroid hormone
PTK	Protein tyrosine kinase
RAAS	Renin angiotensin aldosterone system
RAR	Retinoic acid receptor
RBCs	Red blood cells
RIA	Radioimmunoassay
RNA	Ribonucleic acid
ROS	Reactive oxygen species
R-SMAD	Receptor-regulated SMADs
rT3	Reverse T3
RXR	Retinoic acid X receptor
Ser-Thr	Serine-threonine
SF	Scatter factor
SGLT	Sodium-dependent glucose transporter
SNS	Sympathetic nervous system
T3	Triiodothyronine
T4	Tetraiodothyronine/thyroxine
TBG	Thyroxine-binding globulin
TGF-β	Transforming growth factor-β
TNF-α	Tumor necrosis factor-α
TRH	Thyrotropin releasing hormone
TSH	Thyroid stimulating hormone
VEGF	Vascular endothelial growth factor
VHL	von Hippel-Lindau
VMH	Ventral medial hypothalamus
α-MSH	α-melanocyte-stimulating hormone
β-hCG	β-human chorionic gonadotropin
β-LPH	β-lipotropin

CHAPTER 1

Introduction

Endocrinology is a branch of biology and medicine. The word endocrine means that the secretions of endocrine glands are directly poured into the blood and carried to other parts of the body where they act. The secretions of the endocrine glands are called hormones. It also deals with the disorders of the endocrine system and disease states which arise either due to deficiency or excess of hormones. However, now we know that hormones are also produced by many other organs and tissues which are not endocrine and also act where they are produced. The following terms have therefore been included:

- Autocrine: Hormone binds to autocrine receptors on the same cell by which it has been produced
- Paracrine: Hormone produced by a cell acts on nearby cells. Paracrine hormones diffuse only a short distance, e.g., the somatostatin produced by δ-cells of islet of Langerhans blocks the secretion of both insulin and glucagon from adjacent β-cells and α-cells, respectively. Many cytokines produced by cells of the immune system act in a paracrine manner
- Juxtacrine: Hormone produced by a cell acts on an adjacent cell which is in its direct contact.

HISTORICAL

The history of the development of endocrinology is at least 2,500 years old. In 400 BC, Greek physician, Hippocrates, brought forward the humoral hypothesis. In 200 BC, Aristotle, the Greek philosopher and scientist, noted that prepubertal removal of testes in humans led to short stature, long arms, no growth of facial hair, and change in voice. Around the same time, Chinese scientists started isolating sex and pituitary hormones from urine for medical purposes. Avicenna (980–1,037 AD) in Medieval Persia provided a detailed account of diabetes mellitus in the book "Canon of Medicine". In the 12th century, a description of Graves' disease was given by Dr Al-Jurjani who noted an association of goiter and exophthalmia (protusion of eyes). This disease has been named after Irish physician Robert James Graves. In 1849, Arnold Berthold carried out the experiments where he showed that castrated male cockerels do not develop combs and Wattles and replacement of testes in the abdominal cavity of these or other castrated birds leads to development of combs and wattles. He argued that testes produced some factors that through blood acted in the body of castrated birds to cause these changes. He further showed that an extract of testes has the same effect. Arnold Berthold has been called pioneer of endocrinology. Thomas Addison in 1855 gave the first description of Addison's disease.

In 1902, William Bayliss and Ernest Starling carried out experiments wherein they instilled acid from stomach into the duodenum which caused the secretion of bicarbonate from pancreas to neutralize the acid. They further observed that injecting an extract of jejunal mucosa into the jugular vein had the same effect. They argued that some factor in mucosa was responsible for this effect. They called this factor "secretin". The term hormone was coined for the chemical substances that act in this way. The first gastrointestinal hormone was thus discovered. The same year (1902), epinephrine was purified from adrenal medulla and synthesized in 1904. Prior to this, Joseph Von Mering and Oskar Minkowski in 1889 had shown that the pancreas removed surgically in a dog resulted to an increase in blood and urine glucose (diabetes mellitus). Banting and Best in 1921 injected the homogenate of pancreas into pancreatectomized dogs and showed that the condition can be reversed. Insulin was discovered and was the first peptide hormone to be sequenced by Fredrick Sanger in 1953. After these studies, further researches were carried out to find out how hormones act and now various aspects of endocrinology have been unfolded, and some of which are described in the chapter.

ENDOCRINE GLANDS AND THEIR HORMONES

A detailed list of endocrine glands and their hormones has been mentioned in table 1.1.

TABLE 1.1: Endocrine glands and hormones secreted

Glands	Hormones
1. Pineal gland	• Melatonin • Somatostatin • Norepinephrine • Serotonin
2. Hypothalamus	• Thyrotropin releasing hormone • Gonadotropin releasing hormone • Corticotropin releasing hormone • Growth hormone releasing hormone • Growth hormone release inhibiting hormone/somatostatin • Prolactin release inhibiting hormone • Dopamine

Continued

Continued

3. Pituitary	
a. Anterior pituitary	- Growth hormone - Prolactin - Preopiomelanocortin (it is precursor of at least 10 hormones)/adrenocorticotropic hormone - Thyroid stimulating hormone - Follicle stimulating hormone - Luteinizing hormone
b. Posterior pituitary	- Oxytocin - Vasopressin (antidiuretic hormone)
c. Intermediate pituitary	- Melanocyte stimulating hormone (in humans, intermediate lobe is rudimentary)
4. Thyroid	- Triiodothyronine (T3) - Tetraiodothyronine/thyroxine (T4) - Calcitonin
5. Parathyroid	- Parathormone (Collip's hormone)
6. Pancreas	- Insulin - Glucagon - Somatostatin - Pancreatic polypeptide - Amylin
7. Adrenal	
a. Adrenal cortex	- Aldosterone (secreted by zona glomerulosa) - Cortisol, corticosterone (secreted by zona fasciculata) - Dehydroepiandrosterone, androstenedione (secreted by zona reticularis)
b. Adrenal medulla	- Epinephrine (adrenaline) - Norepinephrine (noradrenaline)

Continued

Continued

8. Gonads	
a. Testis	• Androgens (testosterone, dihydrotestosterone)
b. Ovaries	• Estrogens (estrone, estradiol, estriol) • Progesterone (in corpus luteum)
9. Placenta	• Progesterone, human chorionic gonadotropin, human placental lactogen, inhibin
10. Endothelium	• Nitric oxide
Other endocrine glands and their hormones	
11. Heart	• Atrial natriuretic peptide, brain natriuretic peptide
12. Liver	• Insulin-like growth factor
13. Kidney	• Erythropoietin, renin, vitamin D3(calcitriol), thrombopoietin
14. Adipose tissue	• Leptin, adiponectin, resistin, apelin, visfatin, omentin, asprosin
15. Gastro-intestinal tract	• Gastrin, cholecystokinin, secretin, glucagon, vasoactive intestinal peptide, gastric inhibitory peptide, somatostatin, motilin, ghrelin, gastrin releasing peptide, glucagon-like peptides 1 and 2, peptide YY

Biomolecules that are also considered hormones are retinoic acid and eicosanoids (prostaglandins). Prostaglandins are derived from arachidonic acid, an unsaturated 20-carbon fatty acid with four double bonds.

CHEMICAL NATURE OF HORMONES

Hormones have diverse chemical nature. Vertebrate hormones fall into following chemical classes:

- Derivatives of aromatic amino acids: These are adrenaline (epinephrine), noradrenaline (norepinephrine), dopamine, and thyroid hormones namely triiodothyronine (T3), tetraiodothyronine (T4), and melatonin
- Peptide hormones: These are small in size and have less than 10 amino acid residues, e.g., thyrotropin releasing hormone (TRH), oxytocin, and vasopressin. Thyrotropin releasing hormone is the smallest hormone and is formed of only three amino acid residues
- Polypeptide and protein hormones: These hormones have more than ten amino acid residues, e.g., glucagon, insulin, growth hormone, and parathyroid hormone (PTH). Some protein hormones are formed of more than 100 amino acids residues. The hormones, leptin and adiponectin, produced in white adipose tissue are formed of 167 and 244 amino acids, respectively. Erythropoietin produced in the kidney has molecular weight of 34 Kd
- Glycoprotein hormones: Some polypeptide hormones have carbohydrate (oligosaccharide) side chains attached to them. These are thyroid stimulating hormone (TSH), luteinizing hormone (LH), follicle stimulating hormone (FSH), human chorionic gonadotropin (hCG), α-fetoprotein, inhibin, and erythropoietin. Except erythropoietin, these hormones are formed of two polypeptide units namely, α- and β-subunits. The α-subunits of LH, TSH, and hCG are identical and contain 92 amino acid residues. The β-subunits vary in structure and number of amino acid residues and are responsible for biological function and interaction with their specific receptors, e.g., FSH has a β-subunit of 111 amino acid residues and TSH of 118 amino acid residues. Specific antibodies of these hormones are produced using β-subunits as an antigen. Inhibin is also formed of two chains, α and β. In fact, there are two types of inhibin, which are inhibin A and inhibin B.

Their α-subunit is same but β-subunit is different. α- and β-subunits are linked with each other by a disulphide bond. Activin is also formed of two chains
- Lipid and phospholipid-derived hormones:
    - Steroid hormones: These are derived from cholesterol. All the hormones of adrenal cortex, gonads (testes and ovaries) are steroid hormones. Some hormones of placenta are also steroid hormones
    - Sterol hormone, such as calcitriol (active form of vitamin D), is synthesized from vitamin D
    - Prostaglandins are derived from arachidonic acid
    - Retinoic acid (vitamin A) is a derivative of β-carotene
- Nitric oxide: The only nonorganic hormone synthesized in the endothelium (inner membrane) of blood vessels.

HORMONE CLASSIFICATION BASED ON SOLUBILITY

On the basis of solubility, hormones can be classified into following two main categories.

Group I Hormones

These hormones are lipophilic. As these are insoluble in plasma, they require plasma carrier proteins for their transport. These hormones are inactive when bound to the carrier protein. Only the free hormone is biologically active which can easily traverse the plasma membrane of target cell. These hormones bind with their cognate receptors either in the cytoplasm or in the nucleus. The hormone receptor complex so formed is considered to be the intracellular receptor which binds to the appropriate response element on the genomic deoxyribonucleic acid (DNA) to trigger the transcription of the concerned gene.

Group II Hormones

These hormones are water-soluble, and are thus, easily soluble in the plasma. These combine with extracellular receptors on the plasma membrane of the target cells. Hormone receptor complex so formed triggers the generation of second messengers which communicate with the cell interior. These hormones can be further classified on the basis of type of second messenger used.

- Group II A [using cyclic adenosine monophosphate (cAMP)] [adrenocorticotropic hormone (ACTH), antidiuretic hormone (ADH), PTH, TSH, glucagon]
- Group II B [using cyclic guanosine monophosphate (cGMP)] [atrial natriuretic peptide (ANP), nitric oxide]
- Group II C (using calcium or phosphatidylinositol or both) (acetylcholine, TRH)
- Group II D (using kinase of phosphate cascade) (growth factors, insulin)

Table 1.2 differentiates the two groups of hormones.

TABLE 1.2: Differences between group I and II hormones

	Group I hormones	Group II hormones
Nature	Lipophilic	Hydrophilic
Carrier proteins	Yes	No
Receptor	Intracellular (cytoplasmic or nuclear)	Extracellular
Half-life in plasma	Long (due to protein binding)	Short
Mediator	Hormone receptor complexes	Second messengers (cAMP, cGMP, Ca^{2+}, kinase cascades, phosphatidylinositol metabolites)

Continued

Continued

	Group I hormones	Group II hormones
Examples	Steroid hormones, iodothyronines, calcitriol *	Proteins, polypeptides or catecholamines

cAMP, cyclic adenosine monophosphate; cGMP, cyclic guanosine monophosphate.

*Growth hormone and erythropoietin do not produce second messengers. Their mechanism of action is completely different than other polypeptide and protein hormones (see mechanism of action of growth hormone).

HORMONE AFFINITY

In the extracellular fluid, hormones are present in very low concentration (10^{-15} to 10^{-9} mol/L). This concentration is much lower than the concentration of many structural similar molecules, e.g., peptides, proteins, or amino acids. The hormones have high affinity with their target receptors as the latter not only distinguish different hormones but also a given hormone with 100 fold excess of other similar molecules.

Hormone affinity reflects stability of binding which can be defined by dissociation constant. Hormone binds to receptor to form hormone receptor complex. This complex can dissociate to release free hormone and free receptor. At equilibrium, the rate of the forward reaction becomes equal to that of backward reaction.

$$H + R \underset{k_2}{\overset{k_1}{\rightleftharpoons}} HR$$

The rate constant for the forward (k_1) and backward (k_2) reaction can be combined to define state of these molecules at equilibrium as shown below.

$$k_1 [H][R] = k_1 [HR]$$

The above equation can be rearranged to define dissociation constant Kd. The latter is affinity of hormone with its receptor.

$$\frac{[H][R]}{[HR]} = \frac{k_2}{k_1} = K_d$$

Lower the value of K_d, higher is the affinity and vice versa. K_d can also be defined as the concentration of hormone at which half of the total receptors are bound to the hormone.

PREPROHORMONES

Many hormones are synthesized as preprohormones and cleaved into active form of the hormone. These prehormones contain a presequence which usually functions as a signal peptide and specifies its insertion into or through membranes and help in their secretion. Prosequence plays a crucial role in proper folding of the protein hormone. The following hormones are synthesized as preprohormones.

- Insulin is formed from pre-proinsulin [110 amino acid polypeptide formed of an N-terminal signal peptide and a connecting peptide (C-peptide) which links A and B chain of insulin]. Removal of C-peptide produces mature insulin. Assay of C-peptide is clinically important as its concentration in the circulation is equal to the concentration of insulin produced from the β-cells in the pancreas
- Glucagon is also synthesized as a proglucagon and pancreatic polypeptide (PP) as prepropancreatic polypeptide
- Parathormone as preproparathormone of 115 amino acids. Signal peptide has 25 amino acids. Thus, proparathormone (ProPTH) has 90 amino acids whereas PTH has 84 amino acids
- Preopiomelanocortin is a precursor polypeptide of many hormones. It is formed of 241 amino acid residues. It is synthesized from 285 amino acid precursor pre-proopiomelanocortin by removal of a 44 amino acid signal peptide sequence during translation. It is not a signal peptide. It forms 10 biologically active peptides

- Growth hormone releasing hormone (GHRH) is also formed from a preprohormone. Mature GHRH is formed of 44 amino acids
- Somatostatin is also produced by alternative cleavage of a single preprotein formed of an N-terminal signal peptide
- Angiotensin II, an octapeptide is made from angiotensinogen (having more than 400 amino acids). Angiotensinogen is acted upon by enzyme renin to produce a decapeptide, angiotensin I. Later, removal of two carboxyl terminal amino acids from this decapeptide occurs in lung, epithelial cells, or plasma to form angiotensin II
- Calcitonin is produced by the cleavage of the larger prepropeptide (product of CALC1 gene)
- Gonadotropin releasing hormone (GnRH) is synthesized from a 92-amino acid preprohormone. The final product has 10 amino acids
- Corticotropin releasing hormone (CRH) is 41 amino acid peptide derived from 196 amino acid preprohormone. It is also produced by T-thymocytes and placenta
- Mature ANP is formed of 26 amino acids. It is formed from 151 amino acid preproANP. The latter has a 25 amino acid N-terminal peptide
- Ghrelin is a gastrointestinal hormone (GIT) hormone synthesized as a preprohormone of 117 amino acids. Mature hormone has 28 amino acids. Many other hormones of GIT are also synthesized as preprohormones.

NEGATIVE FEEDBACK CONTROL OF HORMONE LEVELS

Normal physiological hormone levels in blood are maintained by a number of homeostatic mechanisms that require precise signaling between the hormone producing glands and target tissue. This often involves one or more intermediate glands. The best example is hypothalamus pituitary target gland system. The thyroid gland is part of the hypothalamic-pituitary-thyroid axis and control of thyroid hormone secretion is exerted by classical negative feedback (Fig. 1.1). Thyrotropin releasing hormone (also called TRF) from the hypothalamus stimulates thyroid hormone release via TSH secreted from pituitary. As circulating concentrations of thyroid hormones increase, they inhibit both TSH and TRH release. This leads to shutdown of thyroid epithelial cells. Later as circulating levels of thyroid hormones come down, the negative feedback signal fades and release of thyroid hormones becomes normal.

Similarly, GH release is under negative feedback control. Its increased circulating levels inhibit release of GHRH from pituitary and somatostatin from hypothalamus.

Hormones of adrenal cortex are also under negative feedback control. Corticotropin releasing factor (CRF) stimulates adenohypophysis to release ACTH which stimulates

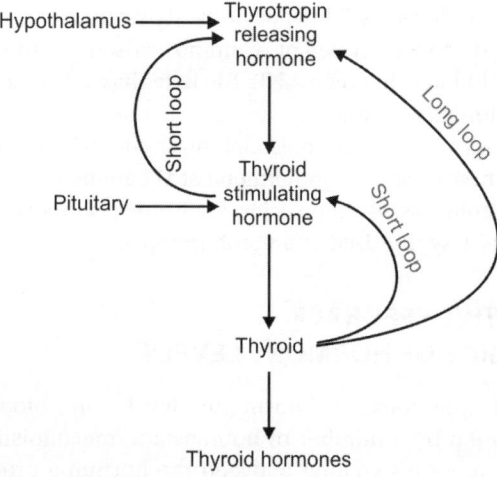

FIG. 1.1: Feedback inhibition

the release of adrenocortical hormones from adrenal cortex. Adrenocorticotropic hormone inhibits the release of CRF and adrenal steroids inhibit the release of both CRF and ACTH.

Pituitary FSH is also under negative feedback control of inhibin, both in males and females. Target gland hormone can either inhibit release of tropic hormone from pituitary (short loop) or releasing hormone from hypothalamus (long loop). Tropic hormone itself can also inhibit release of releasing hormone (short loop).

Some metabolites can also exert negative feedback regulation, e.g., increased blood glucose level (hyperglycemia) causes measured release of insulin from β-cells of islet of Langerhans to increase uptake and utilization of glucose, thereby decreasing blood glucose level, and in turn, diminishing insulin release. Similarly, low blood glucose level (hypoglycemia) causes the release of anti-insulin hormones catecholamines; glucagon, growth hormone, and ACTH which act in various ways to increase blood glucose levels (see also hypoglycemia).

POSITIVE FEEDBACK CONTROL

Some hormones exert positive feedback control. Steroid hormones, estrogen and progesterone, are required for the acute burst of LH secretion that results in ovulation and follicular luteinization and for the further production of these two steroid hormones.

HORMONE ASSAYS

There are many methods to assay hormones. Prior to the discovery of radioimmunoassay technique, hormones were measured depending upon their biological activity. These assays were called bioassays. These are of two types:
1. *In vivo*
2. *In vitro*

In vivo Assay of Insulin

The best example of *in vivo* assays is the effect of insulin on the measurement of blood glucose levels in rabbits. Insulin is injected either intravenously or subcutaneously in an overnight fasted 2 kg rabbit after withdrawing the fasting sample. Glucose level is measured before injection and 2 hours after the injection. That amount of insulin is equivalent to 1 unit of insulin which brings down blood glucose level from 120 to 80 mg/dL of blood. This test can be also done up to a period of 5 hours taking blood samples every hour. The standard insulin and test sample can be compared in this way.

In vitro Assay of Insulin

Rat Hemidiaphragm Assay

Diaphragms are dissected out from overnight fasted male albino rats and kept in chilled buffer solution (balanced salt solution). The diaphragms are then cut into approximately equal halves excluding the posterior tendon and trimmed to remove rough edges and any connective tissue. The hemi-diaphragms after blotting to remove excess fluid are transferred to Warburg flask containing the incubation medium (Krebs's Ringer bicarbonate buffer containing 300 mg glucose per dL). The flasks are gassed for 5 minutes with 95% oxygen and 5% carbon dioxide. Incubation is carried out at 37°C for 90 minutes at the rate of 110–120 oscillations per minute in a shaking water bath. At the end of incubation period, diaphragms are removed and incubation medium analyzed for glucose. The utilization of glucose will be more in the flasks containing insulin than those without insulin. Test insulin, thus, can be calculated in comparison to standard insulin.

Epididymal Fat Pad Assay

This assay is also carried out similar to diaphragm method. Here, the ability of insulin to increase carbon dioxide production from glucose by the fat pad is taken as the parameter for the measurement of the potency of insulin preparation.

Radioimmunoassay

In the word, radioimmunoassay (RIA), radio pertains to radioactive and immuno means antigen-antibody reaction. In this technique, a trace amount of radiolabeled antigen is reacted with its specific antibody. In the presence of unlabeled antigen (standard or test), there is a competition between the labeled antigen and unlabeled antigen for binding sites on the antibody. Higher the concentration of unlabeled antigen, less is the binding of labeled antigen to the antibody. Thus, a standard curve can be drawn by using different concentration of standard antigen (Fig. 1.2). From the standard curve, concentration of the test can be deduced.

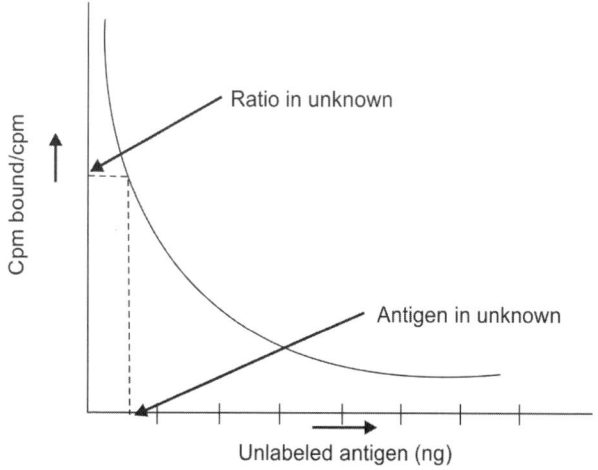

FIG. 1.2: Standard curve radioimmunoassay

This is an extremely sensitive and specific technique because antibodies are specific in nature. It can measure antigens in body fluids (blood) in nanogram and picogram quantities, the concentration at which hormones are present.

This technique was devised in 1956 and published in 1960 by Rosalyn S Yalow and SA Berson for insulin. Rosalyn S Yalow was awarded Nobel Prize in 1977.

Procedure

Antigens are labeled with iodine-125 (^{125}I) (because of its short half-life of about 8 days) using chloramine-T as an oxidizing agent. The ^{125}I binds to tyrosine residues on the polypeptide hormones. Those polypeptides which do not have tyrosine in their structure, tyrosine can be conjugated to those. Antibodies are usually produced in animals like guinea pigs, rabbits, goat, or sheep. The amount of antibody used is such that it binds about 50–60% of the radiolabeled antigen. After incubating the reactants (Ag$^+$ + Ag + antibody; Ag, antigen) in a buffer for a certain period, the antibody bound and free radiolabeled antigen are separated and one of these is counted in a γ-counter and percentage bound is calculated. From this, the amount of test antigen can be calculated. At present, this technique is being used least because of the hazards of radioactivity and involvement of very costly equipment. It still remains important in assay of some hormones such as free T3 and T4. Enzyme-linked immunosorbent assay (ELISA) has almost replaced this technique.

Enzyme-linked Immunosorbent Assay

Enzyme-linked immunosorbent assay is also antigen-antibody reaction dependent method. In ELISA, tracer is an enzyme conjugated antibody rather than radiolabeled antigen. This enzyme linked antibody binds to the antigen. More the antigen present in the test sample, more of this antibody will bind to the antigen. When the substrate is added to this antigen-antibody complex, color is produced. Its absorbance is measured in an ELISA reader. As in radioimmunoassay, the concentration of the antigen in the test sample is calculated from the standard curve drawn by taking different concentrations of the antigen. This assay is carried out in 96 well plates which are polystyrene coated and antigen binds to it. There are various ways ELISA can be performed:

- Indirect ELISA
- Sandwich ELISA
- Competitive ELISA.

There are three enzymes which can be conjugated to the antibody namely:
1. Alkaline phosphatase
2. Horseradish peroxidase (HRP)
3. Beta-D-galactosidase

Chemiluminiscent Assays

Enzyme-linked immunosorbent assay has been further improved by using substrates which produce light (luminescence) rather than colored product. This has increased the sensitivity of the assays, thus resulting in the measurement of very low quantities of the hormone as compared to ELISA. The new assay is called chemiluminescent microparicle immunoassay (CMIA). Enzymes used in CMIA are same as in ELISA, e.g., alkaline phosphatase (AP), HRP, and luciferase, etc. Substrates include luminol, acridine esters, isoluminol, luciferin, and AMPPD. These assays are being used for hormones as well as antibodies (anti-thyroid peroxidase), cancer markers

(CA125), vitamin D3 and drugs and their metabolites. Readymade kits are available and the assays have been fully automatized. These assays have been further modified and one form has been called bidirectionally interfaced chemiluminiscent assay and is used to measure cortisol, FSH, prolactin, testosterone, etc.

Analytical methods include:
- High-performance liquid chromatography for catecholamines—epinephrine, norepinephrine, dopamine, and glycosylated hemoglobin
- Mass spectrometry for 17-OH progesterone and androstenedione.

CHAPTER 2

Hormone Receptors

Hormone receptors are specific molecules that bind a specific hormone. Receptors bind hormones with high affinity as the circulating concentration of hormones is very low. Receptors are of two types:
1. Plasma membrane receptors: These receptors bind catecholamines, peptide, polypeptide, protein, and glycoprotein hormones as these hormones cannot traverse the plasma membrane because of their hydrophobic nature. These receptors are mostly glycoprotein in nature. Membrane receptors are of further two types and are transmembrane in nature. They are as follows:
   i. G-protein coupled receptors: They have 7-transmembrane domains and are linked to heterotrimeric G-proteins via cytoplasmic domain. G-proteins comprise of three subunits namely α, β, and γ.
   ii. Enzyme coupled receptors:
      - Receptor tyrosine kinases
      - Serine-threonine (Ser-Thr) receptor kinases
      - Guanyl cyclase receptors [for atrial natriuretic peptide (ANP) and nitric oxide (NO)]
      - Cytokine receptor family [growth hormone (GH), prolactin, erythropoietin, etc.]

2. **Intracellular receptors:** Receptors for lipid soluble hormones (steroid, thyroid, vitamin A, and vitamin D) are present in the cytoplasm or nucleus of a target cell and form hormone-receptor complexes that bind to deoxyribonucleic acid (DNA).

G-PROTEIN COUPLED RECEPTORS

They are also called heptohelical, 7-TM, serpentine, and G-protein coupled receptors (GPCRs). Functionally, these are so important that nearly 800 are present in humans. About 4% of the 23,000 genes in humans only code for GPCRs.

Their N-terminal is extramembranous and C-terminal is in the cytosol (Fig. 2.1). The 7-TM helices are more of less uniform in size and are formed of 20–27 amino acid residues but their C-terminal vary widely in length amongst different GPCRs. N-terminal length can vary from 7 to 595 residues and C-terminal from 5 to 230 residues. There are two cysteine residues that form disulphide bonds to stabilize receptor structure.

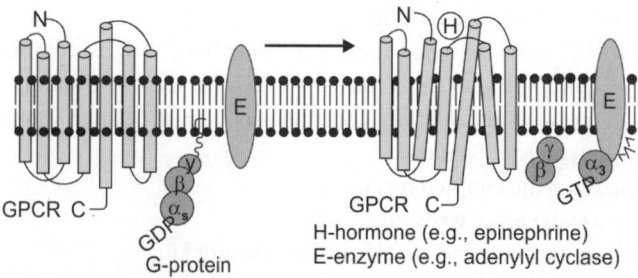

H, hormone (e.g., epinephrine); E, enzyme (e.g., adenylyl cyclase); GPCR, G-protein coupled receptors; GDP, guanosine diphosphate; GTP, guanosine triphosphate.

FIG. 2.1: G-protein coupled receptor

In 2012, Nobel Prize in chemistry was given to Robert Lefkowitz and Brian Kobilka for their work on GPCRs.

RECEPTOR TYROSINE KINASES

Most of these receptors except insulin and insulin-like growth factors (IGFs) receptors are single chain high affinity cell surface receptors. Receptor tyrosine kinases are part of a larger family of protein tyrosine kinases encoded by about 90 genes. Out of these, 58 code only for tyrosine kinases. Each receptor has an extracellular N-terminal ligand binding domain, a hydrophobic transmembrane domain formed of 25–30 amino acids and a C-terminal cytoplasmic domain. This domain is the catalytic domain of the receptor and has the kinase activity. These kinases on ligand binding get autophosphorylated and then phosphorylate their substrates. On ligand binding to the N-terminal extracellular domain, receptor is dimerized with another receptor. Dimerization leads to the activation of cytoplasmic domain and the receptors cross phosphorylate each other and the activated receptor can interact and bind with certain cytoplasmic proteins. The activated receptor may also phosphorylate specific tyrosine residues on a variety of cytoplasmic proteins.

Insulin receptor: It is also a tyrosine kinase receptor. It is formed of 2α and 2β chains joined by disulphide bonds. The α-subunit is composed of 723 amino acids and β-subunit of 620 amino acids. The α-subunit is ligand binding domain and is extracellular whereas β-subunit has an extracellular, transmembrane, and cytoplasmic domain. Cytoplasmic domain has three clusters of tyrosines which are phosphorylated on ligand binding.

Ser-Thr receptor kinases: On ligand binding, these receptors autophosphorylate their serine or threonine residues. Activin, inhibin, and transforming growth factor-β activate these receptors.

Guanyl cyclase receptors: These receptors convert guanosine-5'-triphosphate (GTP) to cyclic guanosine monophosphate (cGMP). These are of two types:
- Membrane bound (for ANP)
- Soluble (for NO).

STEROID AND THYROID HORMONE, VITAMIN A AND VITAMIN D RECEPTORS

Steroid and thyroid hormones, vitamin A and vitamin D are all hydrophobic molecules. They can very easily traverse the plasma membrane. Their receptors, thus, are mostly present in the cytosol or nucleus of the target organs. However, recently some receptors for these hormones have been found on the plasma membrane. These receptors are very large protein molecules (about 100 KDa). These are present in the cytosol or nucleus in an inactive form because some other protein is bound with them [heat shock proteins (HSPs) or corepressor]. On binding the hormone this protein gets separated and the hormone receptor complex becomes active. On binding the hormones, these receptors form dimers either homo or heterodimers. Glucocorticoid receptors are present in the cytoplasm and form homodimers. In the absence of hormones, these are complexed with HSP and are inactive. On ligand binding, HSP is removed and the receptors become active and act as a transcription factor after translocation to the nucleus. The receptors for retinoic acid are present in the nucleus and form heterodimers and are complexed with the corepressor which is removed on ligand binding and the receptor becomes active and acts as transcription factor. Corepressor is a deacetylase which removes acetyl groups from basic amino acids lysine and arginine of histone proteins, thus, preventing

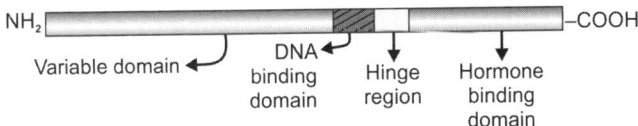

FIG. 2.2: Representation of steroid hormone receptor

them to loosen their grip on DNA. Until and unless DNA opens up transcription will not be initiated.

Steroid hormone receptors are formed of four units called domains (Fig. 2.2):

1. Variable domains: It is the N-terminal part of the receptor and is most variable between the different receptors
2. DNA binding domain: It is present in the center of the receptor. It consists of two nonrepetitive globular motifs in which zinc is coordinated with four zinc fingers. In the nucleus, it binds to hormone response element on the DNA
3. Hinge region: This domain has a nuclear localization signal sequence and helps the receptor to enter nucleus
4. Hormone binding domain: It is present between the central and C-terminal part of the receptor. It can also include nuclear localization sequence, amino acid sequence which can bind chaperones (HSP90 and 60), and parts of dimerization interfaces.

The best characterized steroid receptors are members of the nuclear subfamily 3 (NR3) and include the following:
- Group A: Estrogen receptors α and β
- Group B: Estrogen-related receptors α, β, and γ
- Group C: Ketosteroid receptors
  - Glucocorticoid receptor for cortisol (NR3C1)
  - Mineralocorticoid receptor for aldosterone (NR3C2)
  - Progesterone receptor for progesterone (NR3C3)
  - Androgen receptor for testosterone (NR3C4).

G-PROTEINS (GUANINE NUCLEOTIDE BINDING PROTEINS)

These proteins are a superfamily of GTPases and cleave GTP to guanosine diphosphate (GDP) and phosphate. These are active when bound to GTP and inactive when bound to GDP. On ligand binding, inactive state is converted to active state. The GTPase activity of these proteins again converts active state to inactive by hydrolyzing GTP to GDP + Pi. These are heterotrimeric proteins formed of three subunits α, β, and γ having molecular weight of 45 KDa, 37 KDa and 7 KDa, respectively. It is Gα that binds GDP or GTP. The binding of Gα(GDP)Gβγ to ligand-GPCR complex induces Gα to exchange its bound GDP for GTP. The Gβγ dissociates from Gα and remains associated with very high affinity and dissociates only under denaturing conditions: Both, Gα and Gβγ, are membrane anchored proteins. The Gα is anchored to the inner surface of plasma membrane through either myristic or palmitic acid whereas Gβγ by isoprenylation. Binding of GTP to Gα increases its affinity for adenyl cyclase, thus activating it resulting in the formation of cyclic adenosine monophosphate (cAMP) which acts as a second messenger. The α-subunits of G-proteins are of the following types:

- $G_{S\alpha}$, stimulates adenylate cyclase
- $G_{i\alpha}$, inhibits adenylate cyclase
- $G_{q\alpha}$, activates phospholipase C which produces inositol triphosphate (IP_3) and diacylglycerol (DAG) (see second messengers).

There are many other forms of G protein α-subunits which are activated by other ligand receptor complexes such as odorant receptors, acetylcholine receptors, and rhodopsin receptors.

It is important that active GαGTP is again converted to inactive GαGDP. If GTP remains bound to Gα, it will continue to activate adenyl cyclase resulting into increased levels of cAMP which can be the cause of disease. Several bacterial toxins contain a subunit that penetrates the plasma membrane of cells and cause a chemical modification of Gsα.GTP and prevents hydrolysis of bound GTP to GDP. Cholera toxin from bacterium *Vibrio cholerae*, and enterotoxins of certain strains of *Escherichia coli* act in this way on intestinal epithelial cells resulting in increased levels of cAMP leading to loss of electrolytes and water into the intestinal lumen producing watery diarrhea.

Pertussis toxin produced by *Bordetella pertussis* causes a modification of $G_{i\alpha}$ that prevents release of bound GDP, thus locking it in inactive state resulting into the increased cAMP in the epithelial cells of airways promoting loss of fluids, electrolytes, and mucus secretion causing whooping cough.

SECOND MESSENGERS

When a group II hormone (first messenger or ligand) binds to its specific receptor on the plasma membrane, it induces the production or release of small intracellular signaling molecules which are called second messengers that regulate cellular functions. These include cAMP, cGMP, DAG, and IP_3. The other second messengers, calcium and phosphoinositides, are embedded in cellular membrane. Elevated intracellular concentration of one or more second messengers on binding of a hormone to the cell surface receptors causes a rapid alteration in the activity of one or more enzymes or nonenzymatic proteins. For example, a rise in cAMP induces various changes in cell metabolism that differ in different types of human cells. In fact, cAMP was the first second messenger to be discovered by EW Sutherland who showed that epinephrine on binding to target cells increases glycogenolysis not directly but through

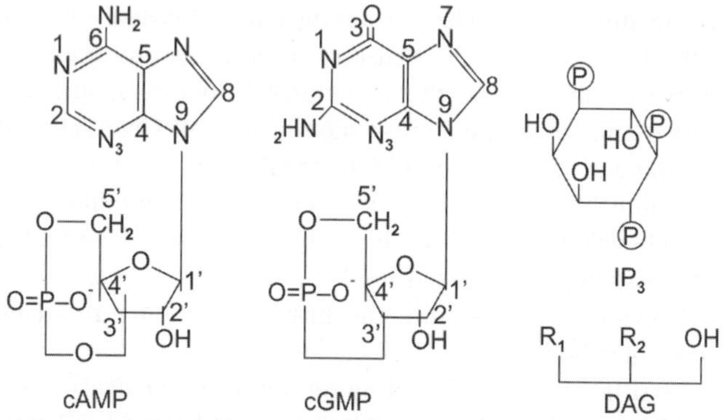

FIG. 2.3: Structure of some second messengers

cAMP, cyclic adenosine monophosphate; cGMP, cyclic guanosine monophosphate; DAG, diacylglycerol; IP3, inositol triphosphate.

elevated levels of cAMP which was formed from adenosine triphosphate by activation of adenyl cyclase through GPCRs. EW Sutherland was awarded Nobel Prize in 1971 for this discovery (Fig. 2.3).

Cyclic guanosine monophosphate is produced by the action of guanyl cyclase. Inositol triphosphate and DAG are produced from phosphoinolitide 4,5 biphosphate present in the plasma membrane by the action of phospholipase C.

As discussed previously, cAMP, cGMP, calcium, IP_3, and DAG are second messengers of hormone signaling. Cyclic adenosine monophosphate is formed through GPCRs. Similarly, cGMP is produced by guanylate cyclase from GTP. Cyclic adenosine monophosphate causes smooth muscle relaxation by stimulating cGMP-dependent protein kinase.

Inositol triphosphate and DAG are produced when a ligand (hormone) binds its receptor and activates a phosphoinositide specific phospholipase C which hydrolyzes phosphoinositide biphosphate (PIP_2) to inositol-1,4,5-

triphosphate (IP_3) and 1,2 DAG. The compound, IP3, is water-soluble whereas DAG is amphipathic. Therefore, IP_3 diffuses through the cytoplasm to endoplasmic reticulum from which it stimulates many cellular processes mainly through calmodulin (calcium binding protein).

Calmodulin is a ubiquitous eukaryotic cytosolic calcium binding dumbbell-shaped 148 amino acid residue monomeric protein. It also occurs as a subunit of larger multimeric protein. It has two globular heads which are connected by a seven turn α-helix. It has two high affinity calcium binding sites in each of its globular heads thus each calmodulin binds 4 calcium ions. These calcium binding sites are formed of nearly superimposable helix-loop-helix motifs called EF hands. On binding calcium, its conformation changes and it activates glycogen phosphorylase kinase and many other calcium regulated proteins, e.g., protein kinase A (PKA).

Glycogen phosphorylase kinase is formed of four subunits (αβγδ). Gamma-subunit (γ-subunit) is the catalytic protein, α- and β-subunits are regulatory subunits which are phosphorylated by PKA and the δ subunit is calmodulin. Phosphorylation of α- and β-subunits increase the affinity of calmodulin for calcium enabling the calcium to bind to the enzyme at the submicromolar calcium concentration. This increases the activity of the enzyme.

Diacylglycerol in the membrane activates a protein kinase C in the presence of calcium and phosphatidylserine. Protein kinase C is capable of activating many enzymes, such as glycogen synthase, by phosphorylating them. It is Ser-The phosphokinase. Diacylglycerol has a steroyl group at C1 and arachidonyl at position 2. In some cells, DAG is degraded by cytosolic phospholipase A to form arachidonate which is a source of eicosanoids, such as prostaglandins, prostacyclin, thromboxane, leukotrienes, and lipoxins, which act as paracrine hormones.

APPLIED ASPECTS

This chapter covers an important area of ligand receptor biochemistry. It is central to understanding which type of receptor is involved in its ligand interaction. Receptors should be construed as check points in biochemical signaling. There can be abundance or paucity of ligand (hormone/transmitter) resulting in well-characterized disorders. For example, in type 1 diabetes mellitus, there is lack of insulin and despite normal or intact insulin receptor, signal transduction is impaired since the receptor cannot be activated. This defect is easily corrected or overcome by supplying ligand (insulin) from outside. Paucity of insulin in circulation can be easily documented by measurement of circulating insulin or c-peptide levels by techniques mentioned earlier. These days, commercially available kits make assays quite easy to undertake and are relatively inexpensive as well.

Now consider a situation where there is no dearth of the ligand (such as insulin), but its receptor is defective. Here again, the ligand-receptor interaction fails to generate (transduce) biochemical signal to affect tissue glucose uptake. Net result again is elevated blood glucose—a hallmark of diabetes mellitus. This situation is encountered where the number and/or affinity of receptor for its ligand is reduced or in rarer situations where the receptor is mutated. This scenario is encountered in type 2 diabetes mellitus. Here, exogenous supply of ligand in usual amounts will not correct the transduction impairment. Large doses would be required to overcome the barrier. Since there are no practical means of replacing a defective receptor, one must resort to other treatment modalities. Receptor number and affinity may be favorably affected in obese patients by weight loss and increased physical activity. In type 2 diabetes mellitus, endogenous insulin levels are increased reflecting a state of insulin resistance. If it were not for insulin resistance (and the receptor signal transduction being intact), we would see persistently low blood glucose (hypoglycemia) as is seen in insulin producing pancreatic islet tumors (insulinoma). High circulating insulin levels with elevated blood glucose imply insulin resistance. High circulating insulin levels with low blood glucose (<50 mg/dL) in the absence of kidney disease call for exclusion of insulinoma. Endocrinologists in academic center can quantitatively measure insulin resistance by technique known as euglycemic-hyperinsulinemic clamp.

Understanding feedback inhibition systems operative in hormone regulation, we have the ability to measure hormones under situations of stimulating or suppressing hormone release, latter being used to test the autonomy of hormone secretion in tumors or hypersecretory states under investigation. When receptor is mutated and signal transduction impaired clinically, the situation is akin to ligand deficiency. It is only through biochemical testing that clear separation of pathogenic mechanisms are sorted out. It has been appreciated for long time that in some situations, alternate or nonclassic ligands may be able to transduce signal.

Biological importance of ligand receptor interaction is better understood via study of signal transduction disorder in some acute and chronic clinical disorders.

Toxin-associated Diseases

- Bacterial endotoxin targeting CD14 surface protein of macrophage leading to secretion of cytokines (including IL-2), generation of reactive oxygen species (ROS), arachidonic acid, and NO
- Cholera toxin targeting GTP-binding protein of intestinal epithelial cells resulting in inappropriately elevated cAMP with consequent loss of electrolytes into the lumen of intestines

- Pertussis toxin targeting GTP-binding proteins of airways epithelial cells
- Domoic acid: Potent agonist of glutamate (N-methyl-D-aspartate) receptor.

Genetic Defects of Plasma Membrane Receptor Interaction or Function

Insulin

- Defective ligand: Abnormal insulin (hormone molecule)
- Defective receptor
  - Reduced receptor number (type A insulin resistance)
  - Insulin receptor antibody (extreme insulin resistance–type B)
  - Reduced receptor affinity (type E insulin resistance)
  - No receptor for insulin (insulin resistance type D)
  - Postbinding defect (insulin resistance type C)
  - Postreceptor defect (insulin resistance type F). Extreme insulin resistance: Leprechaunism.

Growth Hormone

- Defective receptor binding—Laron dwarfism (low IGF-1 generation)

Vasopressin

- Defective receptor binding: Nephrogenic diabetes insipidus

Thyroid

- Activating mutation of thyroid stimulating hormone (TSH) receptor leading to hyperthyroid state
- Mutation of thyroid hormone transporters leading to thyroid hormone resistant state and manifesting as hypothyroidism with features depending on the isoform of thyroid hormone receptor that is affected.

Parathyroid
- Insensitivity to biologic effect of parathyroid hormone.

Adrenocorticotropic Hormone
- Adrenocorticotropic hormone (ACTH) receptor mutation affecting biological effects of ACTH: Familial glucocorticoid deficiency.

Luteinizing Hormone
- Luteinizing hormone receptor mutation: Male precocious puberty.

Genetic Defects of Intracellular Receptor Function
- Androgen receptor mutation: Complete androgen insensitivity or partial insensitivity
- Thyroid hormone (T3) receptor mutation: Thyroid hormone resistance syndrome
- Cortisol receptor mutation: Cortisol resistance, behaving like adrenal insufficiency
- 1, 25 Dihydroxycholecalciferol: Vitamin D resistance:
  - No receptor
  - Reduced receptor number
  - Reduced receptor affinity
  - Defective receptor translocation.

Autoimmune Disease
- Type 1 diabetes mellitus (insulin antibodies, glutamic acid decarboxylase-65 antibodies, zinc transporter 8 antibody)
- Myasthenia gravis (antibodies against acetylcholine receptor)
- Graves' disease: (stimulating TSH receptor antibodies)
- Lambert-Eaton myaesthenic syndrome is a syndrome where antibodies target neuromuscular junction impairing release of acetylcholine leading to muscular weakness and depressed reflexes.

It should be noted that chronic exposure of receptor to its ligand leads to receptor desensitization and thus reduced or impaired signal transduction. Sometimes, this phenomenon is exploited for therapeutic purpose employing long, acting hormone agonists such as in treatment of hormone-dependent endocrine or oncologic disorders (precocious puberty, uterine fibroids, prostate cancer, etc.)

CHAPTER 3

Hypothalamus

In biology, hypo pertains to low or below. Hypothalamus is a portion of the brain located below the thalamus and just above the brainstem. In humans, it is roughly the size of an almond. It synthesizes and secretes a number of neurohormones also called releasing/inhibiting hormones (hypophyseotropic factors) which stimulate or inhibit the secretion of pituitary hormones. It is an extremely important part of diencephalon that is involved in the mediation of autonomic, behavioral, and autonomic functions. It is involved in release/synthesis of 8 major hormones from pituitary, temperature regulation, control of food and water intake, sexual behavior and reproduction, and mediation of emotional response. It is thought to contain "biological clock" that regulates body functions at different times of day or those that vary over period of many days. Lesions of hypothalamus often disrupt sleep-waking cycle. It is the central relay point for coordinating information from multiple inputs and guiding pituitary hormonal response.

- Hypothalamus contains a number of small nuclei which serve many functions
- Medial preoptic nucleus regulates the release of gonadotropic hormones from adenohypophysis

- Supraoptic nucleus. It is a nucleus of magnocellular neurosecretory cells. The cell bodies produce vasopressin also known as antidiuretic hormone
- Paraventricular nucleus affects thyrotropin-releasing hormone, corticotrophin, and oxytocin release
- Anterior hypothalamic nucleus also affects thyrotropin release
- Arcuate nucleus affects growth hormone-releasing hormone release
- Posterior nucleus affects vasopressin release.

Following releasing factors are produced by the hypothalamus:
- Thyrotropin-releasing hormone: This hormone stimulates anterior pituitary to release thyroid stimulating hormone. Thyrotropin-releasing hormone is made up of three amino acids; namely histidine, proline, and pyroglutamate (glutamate derivative)
- Gonadotropin-releasing hormone (GnRH): This hormone is a decapeptide and stimulates anterior pituitary to release luteinizing hormone and follicle-stimulating hormone (gonadotropins)
- Corticotropin-releasing hormone: This hormone stimulates the release of adrenocorticotropic hormone from anterior pituitary. Adrenocorticotropic hormone stimulates adrenal cortex to release its steroid hormones
- Growth hormone-releasing hormone: This hormone stimulates anterior pituitary to release growth hormone also known as somatotropin. Growth hormone-releasing hormone is made up of 44 amino acids
- Growth hormone release-inhibiting hormone: Growth hormone release-inhibiting hormone is also known as *somatostatin* and is made up of 14 amino acids. It inhibits the release of GH from anterior pituitary

- Prolactin release-inhibiting hormone: It is a small peptide and inhibits the release of Prolactin from anterior pituitary
- Prolactin inhibiting hormone (dopamine): It is the primary physiological inhibitor of prolactin secretion. It is the only nonpeptide hypothalamic biochemical which has a specific hypophysiotropic function. By virtue of its dual role as a neurotransmitter and a hormone, it provides the best example of neuroendocrine interactions.

APPLIED ASPECTS

Hypothalamic hormones are commercially available to test integrity of hypothalamus-pituitary axis. Endocrinologists use them routinely to diagnose deficiency of pituitary hormones by studying release or lack thereof of pituitary hormones following injection of hypothalamic hormone(s). This testing is often referred to as dynamic testing. Lack of response is indicative of pituitary hormone deficiency that could be caused by damage to pituitary gland resulting from invasion, infection, infiltration, or inflammation of pituitary gland.

Sometimes, hypothalamic hormones may be produced outside hypothalamus by a variety of tumors driving excess pituitary hormone production leading to pituitary hormone excess states. These tumors are found in different locations outside the hypothalamus pituitary confines (ectopic hormone production). Final confirmation is obtained by immunohistochemical staining of sample obtained from the tumor.

Since somatostatin and dopamine are releasing inhibiting factors, these are used in curtailing secretion of excessive growth hormone or prolactin by pituitary tumors. Long-acting analogs are commercially available for this purpose. Excess production of growth hormone in acromegaly is treated by long-acting analog of somatostatin while excessive production of prolactin by pituitary tumors is effectively treated by long-acting analog of dopamine.

Taking advantage of receptor desensitization following chronic exposure to its ligand, long acting analogs of GnRH have been used to reduce excessive production of gonadotropins in young children to treat premature onset of puberty in children (precocious puberty). This desensitization is reversible once exposure to ligand is discontinued.

CHAPTER 4

Pituitary Gland

Pituitary gland is the master endocrine gland as it controls the working of other endocrine glands in the body. It is itself under the control of hypothalamus. It is divided into anterior pituitary (adenohypophysis) and posterior pituitary (neurohypophysis), intermediate lobe is vestige in humans. It is an important endocrine organ that regulates diverse and interconnected physiological functions such as growth, development, metabolism, reproductive functions, and stress response. This gland measures 15 × 10 × 6 mm and weighs about 500–900 mg. During pregnancy, it nearly triples in size returning to prepregnancy volume during the next few weeks following delivery.

ANTERIOR PITUITARY

The hormones produced by anterior pituitary directly or indirectly influence a variety of biochemical processes. The hormones are broadly classified as:
- Growth hormone-prolactin group
- Pro-opiomelanocortin peptide family
- Glycoprotein hormones.

Growth Hormone-prolactin Group

It includes growth hormone, prolactin, placental lactogen, or chorionic somatomammotropin. These hormones have many structural resemblances.

Growth hormone: It is also called somatotropin and is produced by special acidophilic cells called somatotrophs. Growth hormone is a 191 amino acid single chain polypeptide having molecular weight of around 22,000 Daltons (22 KDa). Growth hormone-releasing hormone and growth hormone release-inhibiting hormone, also known as somatostatin, produced in hypothalamus control the release of growth hormone. Ghrelin, a gut hormone increases growth hormone secretion. The production of growth hormone is influenced by many factors such as sleep, exercise, food intake, pain, and cold.

Growth Hormone-biochemical Functions

- Growth hormone promotes growth and development of the body. Its growth promoting effects are mediated through insulin-like growth factor 1 (IGF-1) also known as somatomedin
- Growth hormone increases protein synthesis in the tissues by the uptake of amino acids. Thus this hormone leads to positive nitrogen balance. It also increases deoxyribonucleic acid and ribonucleic acid synthesis. It decreases urinary excretion of urea
- It causes hyperglycemia by increasing gluconeogenesis, decreasing glucose utilization, and glucose uptake. It also impairs glycolysis in body cells. Thus, its effects are antagonistic to insulin
- Growth hormone increases the concentration of fatty acids in the blood by promoting lipolysis in adipose tissue
- Growth hormone promotes bone growth by promoting its mineralization especially in growing children. In children, it also increases formation of cartilage

Pituitary Gland

- In circulation, its half-life is 30 minutes
- It has a specific binding protein in plasma.

Mechanism of Action

Janus kinase/signal transducers and activators of transcription (JAK-STAT) pathway of signaling: Growth hormone and erythropoietin (produced in kidney) act through JAK-STAT pathway of signaling. Receptors for these hormones are activated through ligand-induced receptor aggregation of two or more receptor components. These receptors have an ectodomain, a transmembrane domain, and a cytosolic domain. The signal is transmitted within the cell by the JAK-STAT pathway after binding of the hormone to their cognate receptors. These receptors form complexes with protein of JAK family of nonreceptor tyrosine kinases, so named because each of the four on 150 amino acid residue members (JAK1, JAK2, JAK3, and Tykq) has two protein tyrosine kinase (PTK) domains. Only its C-terminal domain is functional. Signal transducers and activator of transcription are formed of a family of 700–800 residue proteins. Activation of these transcription factors is regulated by tyrosine phosphorylation.

Janus kinase lack both SH2 and SH3 domains which are present in other tyrosine kinases. For growth hormone and erythropoietin, the receptor subunits are bound as homodimers. Janus kinase activation occurs when ligand mediated receptors form homodimers because two JAKs are brought into close proximity allowing trans-phosphorylation. The activated JAKs phosphorylate STATs. Phosphorylation of STATS permits dimerization of STATS through interaction with a conserved SH2 domain. Phosphorylated STATS enter the nucleus. Within the nucleus, STATs bind specific regulatory sequences to activate transcription of target genes. You will note that though the receptors for growth hormone and erythropoietin are present on the plasma membrane of target cells, the ligand binding does not result in the production of second messengers. Thus, this is a direct mechanism to translate an extracellular signal into a transcriptional response.

Prolactin

It is also called luteotropin or mammotropin or luteotropic hormone. Its structure is like growth hormone. It is a single chain polypeptide of 198 amino acids and has a molecular weight of 22,800 Da. It has three disulphide bonds in its structure. Its role in female physiology is well studied as against the male physiology where its role has not been established with certainty. Circumstances favoring its release resemble those affecting release of adrenocorticotropic hormone (ACTH), a classic stress hormone. Prolactin receptors are found on macrophages, T and B lymphocytes which would argue for its role in immune-competence (immune and endocrine system interaction). Its release is primarily regulated through tonic inhibition by dopamine.

Prolactin-biochemical Functions

- Prolactin stimulates lactose production in mammary glands. It is required for initiation and maintenance of lactation in mammals
- It is called luteotropic hormone as it promotes the growth of corpus luteum which produces progesterone
- Several enzymes of carbohydrate and lipid metabolism are increased by prolactin
- Highly elevated levels of prolactin decrease the levels of estrogen in females and testosterone in males
- Prolactin in male mice enhances luteinizing hormone receptors in Leydig cells resulting in testosterone secretion, which further leads to spermatogenesis. Its relevance in humans is poorly understood.

Pro-opiomelanocortin Peptide Family

A single gene of anterior and intermediate lobe of pituitary is involved in the production of all the members of pro-opiomelanocortin (POMC) family. Pro-opiomelanocortin (made of 241 amino acids) is a single polypeptide that is precursor to multiple hormones. The name pro-opiomelanocortin is given because of the fact that it is prohormone to opioids, melanocyte stimulating hormone, and corticotrophin. The different hormones are produced by a process called differential splicing.

Pro-opiomelanocortin Products

Pro-opiomelanocortin consists of three peptide groups:
1. Adrenocorticotropic hormone which gives rise to α-melanocyte-stimulating hormone (α-MSH) and corticotrophin-like intermediate lobe peptide
2. β-Lipotropin (β-LPH) which produces γ-LPH, β-MSH, and β-endorphin. The latter gives rise to γ- and α-endorphins
3. An N-terminal peptide that forms γ-MSH.

Adrenocorticotropic hormone: This hormone is released from anterior pituitary under the influence of corticotropin-releasing hormone produced in hypothalamus. This hormone is made of 39 amino acids and has a molecular weight of 4500. Its main role is to regulate the secretion of hormones from adrenal cortex (glucocorticoids, mineralocorticoids, sex steroids). In adrenal cortex, it promotes the conversion of cholesterol into pregnenolone and also increases lipolysis.

β-Lipotropin: It is made up of 93 carboxy terminal amino acids of POMC. It is only found in the pituitary and not in other tissues as it is rapidly degraded. It consists of γ-LPH and β-endorphin which give rise to β-MSH and γ-endorphin respectively. Gamma-endorphin forms α-endorphin, which further gives rise to enkephalin as shown in the figure 4.1.

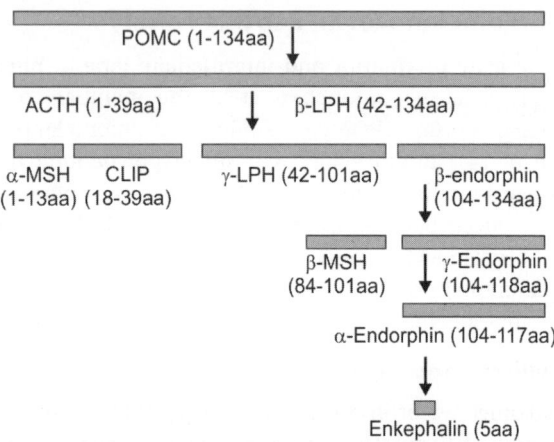

POMC, pro-opiomelanocortin; MSH, melanocyte-stimulating hormone; LPH, lipotropin; CLIP, corticotrophin-like intermediate lobe peptide; ACTH, adrenocorticotropic hormone.

FIG. 4.1: Pro-opiomelanocortin gene products

Beta-endorphin (31aa) gives rise to modified products α-endorphin (15aa) and γ-endorphin (14aa). Alpha-endorphin gives rise to pentapeptide enkephalins. The function of β-LPH is to promote lipolysis and act as precursor (prohormones) for synthesis of β-endorphin and enkephalins (both act as analgesics).

Enkephalins: These are neurotransmitters having opiate like effects on central nervous system and are thus also called opioid-peptides. The word endorphins mean inner morphine (self-opioids). These are penta-peptides. Enkephalins are of two types. These are methionine enkephalin and leucine enkephalin having methionine and leucine as their C-terminal amino acids, respectively.

Melanocyte stimulating hormone: In some animals, α- and β-MSH are functional; while in humans, γ-MSH is more important. The activity of γ-MSH is contained in β-LPH (precursor of γ-MSH) or γ-LPH. Melanocyte-stimulating hormone promotes melanogenesis which leads to skin color darkening in some animals but in humans it does not have any such role.

Glycoprotein Hormones

These include TSH, follicle stimulating hormone (FSH), and luteinizing hormone. The last two are called gonadotropins. Human chorionic gonadotropins is also included in gonadotropins but it is produced by the placenta and not by the pituitary.

Thyroid-stimulating hormone (TSH): It is a glycoprotein hormone formed of an α and a β chain and has a molecular weight of 30 KDa. It is released from the pituitary in response to thyrotropin-releasing hormone. Thyroid-stimulating hormone secretion is under feedback inhibition by T_3 and T_4. Thyroid-stimulating hormone binds to cell surface receptor and stimulates expression of Na^+-I^- symporter allowing transport of Iodide cross concentration gradient. Thyroid-stimulating hormone also enhances the conversion of I^- to I^+. Thyroid-stimulating hormone also promotes proteolysis of thyroglobulin to release T_3 and T_4 into blood circulation.

Gonadotropins: Follicle stimulating hormone and luteinizing hormone are released from anterior pituitary under the influence of gonadotropin-releasing hormone (GnRH) from hypothalamus. Both are glycoprotein hormones formed of an α- and β-chain. The α-chains are identical in structure but β-chains are different. Both have a molecular weight of around 30 kDa. Both chains are required for biological activity but specific antibodies can be produced by using their β-chains as antigens.

Follicle stimulating hormone in females enhances the growth of ovarian follicles and production of estrogen from them. In males, FSH stimulates growth of seminiferous tubules and is required for testosterone production and spermatogenesis. Luteinizing hormone stimulates corpus luteum to secrete progesterone in females and Leydig cells in males to secrete testosterone.

POSTERIOR PITUITARY

Oxytocin and vasopressin or antidiuretic hormone (ADH) nonapeptides synthesized by the hypothalamus and stored in the posterior pituitary. On appropriate stimulation, these are released into the circulation. Each hormone is transported through axons in association with specific carrier proteins called neurophysins I and II, respectively. Vaginal or uterine distension and neural impulses of nipple stimulation cause the release of oxytocin from posterior pituitary. Estrogen also stimulates the production of oxytocin and progesterone inhibits it. In fact estrogen increases responsiveness to oxytocin by increasing expression of oxytocin receptors (OXTR). On the other hand, release of ADH is mostly controlled by osmoreceptors in hypothalamus and baroreceptors of heart. Antidiuretic hormone secretion is stimulated by increase in osmolarity of plasma and/or reduction in effective plasma volume.

Structure of Oxytocin

$$\text{Cys-Tyr-Ile-Gln-Asn-Cys-Pro-Leu-Gly-NH}_2$$
$$\overline{\qquad\text{S-S}\qquad}$$

Oxytocin-biochemical Functions

- Oxytocin causes contraction of uterine smooth muscles and induces labor
- Oxytocin causes contraction of myoepithelial cells of mammary glands to cause milk ejection.

Mechanism of Action of Oxytocin

Its receptor is a G-protein coupled receptors (GPCR) and called OXTR. Its G-protein α-subunit is Gq and activates phospholipase C.

Vasopressin (Antidiuretic Hormone)

It is a nonapeptide containing cysteine at positons 1 and 6 which are linked by a S-S bond (disulphide bridge). The structure of oxytocin and vasopressin differ by two amino acids at position 3 and 8. In oxytocin, isoleucine and leucine are present at position 3 and 8; whereas in vasopressin, phenylalanine and arginine are present at position 3 and 8, respectively (see structure). In some animals, vasopressin has a lysine in place of arginine at position 8.

Structure of Vasopressin

$$Cys-Tyr-Phe-Gln-Asn-Cys-Pro-Arg-Gly-NH_2$$
$$\underline{\qquad\qquad S-S \qquad\qquad}$$

Antidiuretic Hormone-biochemical Functions

- Antidiuretic Hormone helps in the reabsorption of water from nephrons of the kidneys which results in increased blood pressure. Thus, ADH is primarily concerned with the regulation of water balance in the body.

Mechanism of Action of Vasopressin

Vasopressin also acts through GPCRs. It binds to three types of receptors V1, V2, and V3. Receptor V1 is found in high density on the surface of vascular smooth muscle and ligand binding causes vasoconstriction by activating phospholipase C. This receptor is also present on platelets and on stimulation induces an increase in intracellular calcium facilitating thrombosis. In kidney, these receptors are found in high density on medullary interstitial cells, vasa recta, and epithelial cells of the collecting duct. Vasopressin binding to these receptors results in reduced blood flow to inner medulla. These receptors are also present on the luminal membrane of the collecting duct and limit the antidiuretic effect of the hormone.

V2 receptor is different from V1 receptor in a way that it is G-protein α-subunit is Gsα rather than Gqα. It thus activates adenyl cyclase and increases the levels of cyclic adenosine monophosphate. Antidiuretic action of ADH is mediated by V2 receptor. V3 receptor is also a GPCR and activates several signaling pathways via different G-proteins in different tissues depending on receptor density.

Since plasma osmolality and volume primarily determine secretion of arginine vasopressin (AVP), endocrinologists often manipulate intravascular volume or osmolality to study release of AVP in order to study disorders affecting water or sodium metabolism. This is seen often in situations where there is deficiency of AVP encountered in diabetes insipidus resulting in massive water loss and hypernatremia (elevated plasma sodium level). Conversely, water retention and hyponatremia may be seen if there is inappropriate secretion of AVP—a condition known as syndrome of inappropriate antidiuretic hormone (inappropriate secretion of ADH). Since osmolality is critical to cellular function, a change of 2% in osmolality impacts AVP secretion.

PATHOPHYSIOLOGY OF PITUITARY GLAND

Dwarfism/short stature: It is caused by deficiency of growth hormone in children. Patient is dwarf but has well proportionate body. Metabolic defects generally are not serious in nature. Pediatricians monitor growth of babies/children using gender specific growth charts, and make referrals to endocrinologist if a growth disorder is suspected. Those found to growth hormone deficient can be treated very effectively with growth hormone replacement.

Gigantism: Excessive production of growth hormone in children leads to rapid longitudinal growth. This may be due to acidophil tumor in the pituitary gland. Increase in the length of long bones occurs before the closure of epiphyseal plates. Symptoms include headaches, increase in the size of hands and feet. There is excessive body hair growth, and the skin may appear oily. Diagnosis is made by documenting increase in circulating growth hormone and IGF-1 levels. This is confirmed by failure to suppress growth hormone levels following a glucose load.

Acromegaly: It is caused by excessive production of growth hormone in adults. There is no increase in the length of bones after closure of epiphyseal plate. Symptoms include increase in the size of hands and face. Skin gets thickened and there is excessive hair growth on the body. Diagnosis is made by documenting increased circulating levels of growth hormone and IGF-1. Failure to suppress growth hormone level following a glucose load serves as the confirmatory test. These days surgery is the first treatment of choice. Alternatively, somatostatin analog (long acting) may be used if surgery is not feasible or if surgery has failed. Growth hormone receptor antagonist is also in use.

Cushing's disease: It refers to excessive production of ACTH by a pituitary tumor leading to excessive cortisol production from the adrenal glands. Patients have central obesity, hypertension, proximal muscle weakness, and thinning of skin leading to easy bruisability. Patients have elevated blood glucose and abnormal lipid profile. Women in pre-menopausal years have menstrual irregularity. Diagnosis is made by documenting high plasma cortisol level with concurrent inappropriately normal ACTH levels.

Gonadotroph adenoma: Tumors secreting luteinizing hormone and FSH are common in adults and mostly clinically silent.

However, during early childhood they may lead to early initiation of puberty—precocious puberty. Gonadotropin-releasing hormone receptor desensitization using long acting GnRH agonists have been effectively used to treat this condition.

Diabetes insipidus: This disease is caused by deficiency of ADH arising from damage to hypothalamus (central diabetes insipidus). This results in decreased water reabsorption from nephrons of kidney. As a result dilute urine is produced with concurrent increase plasma osmolality. Serum sodium levels are high and patient is at high risk for dehydration. It is a life-threatening condition if left untreated. It is differentiated from decompensated diabetes mellitus by absence of glucose in urine. Treatment rests on replacement of water and provision of AVP (given as desmopressin). Milder forms may require water replacement and adequate hydration only.

APPLIED ASPECTS

Pituitary gland is central to all endocrine axes and its functional integrity is vital to all functions relating to growth, development, sexual differentiation, reproduction, and adaptation to environmental stress. Pituitary modulates hormone secretion depending on the developmental stages of life and operates under a very sensitive negative feedback and feed forward system. It is subject to assault by inflammation/infection, infiltration, infarction/bleeding and developmental abnormalities. When pituitary cells are damaged, hormone production is drastically reduced depending on the cell type(s) damaged. In order to test the integrity of cell, commercially available trophic factors from the hypothalamus or the standard stimuli known to cause release of pituitary hormone can be used to assess pituitary function—these are often referred to as dynamic tests.

On the other hand, if there is an autonomous transformation of a particular hormone secreting cell type resulting in excessive production of hormone. Hormone normally produced by the distal target gland is used to see if pituitary responds by significantly reducing its hormone output (normal response). This kind of testing allows targeting treatment at the site of defect. These tests are known as suppression tests.

Hormone replacement in deficient states is easy, relatively cheap, and effective. Prolactin secreting tumors respond favorably to medical therapy—dopamine agonists. All other pituitary tumors would be offered surgery as the first mode of treatment.

CHAPTER 5

Thyroid Gland

Thyroid gland is located at the front of the neck below larynx on either side of trachea. It weighs about 25 g in an adult. It is the largest endocrine gland having two lobes connected by isthmus. This gland produces triiodothyronine (T3), thyroxine (T4), and calcitonin. In the connective tissue between thyroid follicles, C-cells are present which are source of the hormone calcitonin that helps in regulation of calcium levels. Among all endocrine glands, this gland is most susceptible to hypo- or hyperfunction. Thyroid hormones are derivatives of amino acid tyrosine. They are most like amine or peptide in structure, but more like steroid hormones in solubility and activity. Approximately, 100 µg of thyroid hormones are secreted each day from the gland principally in the form of T4 and about 10% as T3, and smaller amount as reverse T3 (rT3).

TRIIODOTHYRONINE AND THYROXINE

- Both these diamino acids are derivatives of tyrosine
- Both require rare element iodine for bioactivity
- Both are synthesized as a part of precursor molecule thyroglobulin
- T3 is more active and largely (80%) derived from T4 by deiodination in peripheral tissues

- T4: T3 ratio is 7:1 when iodine is in sufficient supply
- Thyroglobulin (Molecular mass of 660 kDa) is a large iodinated and glycosylated protein having 8-10% carbohydrate content and is the precursor of T3 and T4
- On stimulation by thyroid-stimulating hormone (TSH), thyroglobulin present in the colloid is internalized into thyroid follicular cells. After hydrolysis by proteases and peptidases (lysosomal enzymes), T3 and T4 are released from basal portion of thyroid follicular cells into the blood.

STRUCTURE OF THYROID HORMONES

BIOSYNTHESIS OF THYROID HORMONES

- Iodide (I$^-$) is transported into thyroid follicular cells against concentration gradient by using Na$^+$/I$^-$ symporter regulated by the TSH. Iodide is 25 times more in thyroid gland than in serum. The Na$^+$/K$^+$ ATPase dependent channel returns sodium back into serum. Thyroid-stimulating hormone is a complex glycoprotein that interacts with a G-protein linked thyroid membrane cell surface receptor. There are approximately 1,000 TSH receptors on the basal surface of each thyroid follicular cell

- Iodide ion is then oxidized into I⁺ in the presence of heme containing peroxidase utilizing H_2O_2. This step is essential for iodide organification and synthesis of T3 and T4. Hydrogen peroxide is made available by a nicotinamide adenine dinucleotide phosphate-dependent enzyme
- Oxidized iodide (I⁺) combines with tyrosyl residues on thyroglobulin to form monoiodothyronine (MIT) and di-iodothyronine (DIT). This process is called iodination. The 3rd position of aromatic ring is iodinated first followed by iodination of 5th position. Once iodination occurs, the iodine cannot easily leave the thyroid gland
- In the next step called coupling, two DIT molecules combine to form T4 and MIT and DIT molecules combine to form T3. This reaction seems to be catalyzed by the same peroxidase by stimulating free radical formation. This step occurs within the thyroglobulin molecule. Thyroglobulin is a secretory protein and its biosynthesis starts in the rough endoplasmic reticulum where its glycosylation is initiated
- Thyroglobulin is then internalized into thyroid follicular cells by pinocytosis and phagocytosis. Here it fuses with lysosomes. The proteases and peptidases of lysosomes hydrolyze thyroglobulin to release T3 and T4 into the blood. Monoiodothyronine and DIT are also released
- Monoiodothyronine and DIT are then deiodinated to release iodide which is reused in the thyroid. Deiodination of T4 into T3 largely occurs outside the thyroid gland in the peripheral tissues (extrathyroidal deiodination).

The sequence of events is shown in figure 5.1.

Transport of Triiodothyronine and Thyroxine

Most of the thyroid hormones circulate in the plasma bound to specific proteins namely:
- Thyroxine-binding globulin (TBG): It is a glycoprotein which binds T3 and T4 with 100 times affinity than thyroxine-binding prealbumin. It binds to nearly all the T3

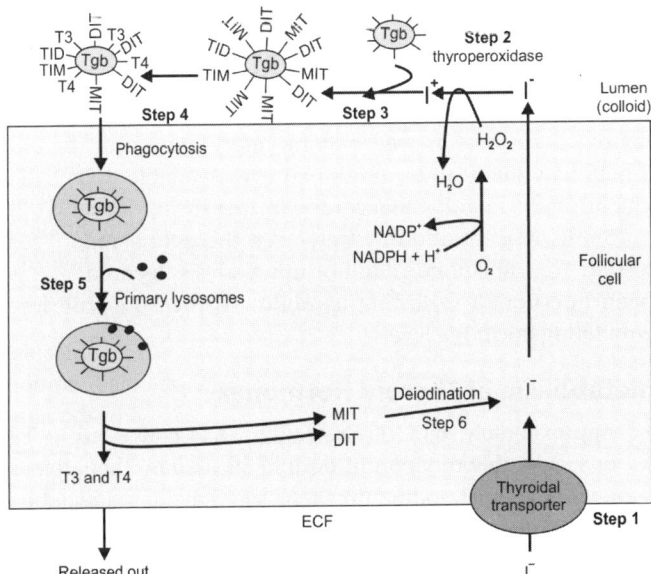

ECF, extracellular fluid; MIT, monoiodothyronine; DIT, diiodothyronine; NADP, nicotinamide adenine dinucleotide phosphate.

FIG. 5.1: Thyroid hormone biosynthesis

and T4 noncovalently. This protein is produced in the liver and its synthesis is increased by estrogens (present in birth control pills). Conversely, androgens reduce concentration of TBG. Thyroxine-binding globulin is a high affinity low binding capacity protein. It binds 70% of T4 and 80% of T3
- Thyroxine-binding prealbumin: Transthyretin.
- Albumin: It is low affinity and high capacity binding protein, and binds 20% of T4 and T3.

When thyroid hormones are in bound form, they are not active. That is why estimation of total T3 and T4 can be misleading since binding protein concentration may change during acute illness. Free T3 (0.3%) and free T4 (0.03%) are biologically active and hence their measurement is of great diagnostic value. It should be noted that not only are the binding protein concentrations impacted during severe illness, there may be impact of clearance and degradation of thyroid hormones as well making interpretation of thyroid functions difficult to an untrained eye. Available diagnostic kits are notorious for inaccuracy in measuring free thyroid hormone concentrations. Lately even the gold standard for testing free hormone, equilibrium dialysis technique has been questioned regarding its ability to measure true free circulating hormone levels.

Metabolism of Thyroid Hormones

- Approximately, 80% of circulating T4 is converted to T3 or rT3 by deiodination in peripheral tissues. The latter is a weak agonist. Iodine thus released may be reutilized by thyroid gland. Thyroid hormones may undergo inactivation by total deiodination, deamination, and decarboxylation. Deamination produces tetraiodothyroacetic acid (from T4) and tri-iodothyroacetic acid (from T3)
- In the liver, thyroid hormones may undergo glucuronidation and sulfation making them more hydrophilic
- These hydrophilic metabolites may be excreted into the bile, deiodinated in the kidney or excreted in the urine as glucuronide conjugate.

Biochemical Functions of Thyroid Hormones

- They increased basal metabolic rate of the body by stimulating metabolism and increasing oxygen consumption in many body tissues except brain, testes, lungs, and retina. Thyroid hormones increase the activity of Na^+/K^+ ATPase which increases heat production in the body. They increase the size and number of mitochondria

- Thyroid hormones promote protein synthesis by acting like steroid hormones and activating deoxyribonucleic acid (DNA). They thus cause positive nitrogen balance and promote growth and development of the body
- They cause hyperglycemia by promoting gluconeogenesis and glycogenolysis. They also promote intestinal glucose absorption
- They stimulate lipid utilization and thus have hypolipidemic effects
- Thyroid hormones are required for metamorphosis of tadpole into frog. During metamorphosis, there is resorption of tail, epidermal changes, stimulation of urea cycle enzymes etc.
- A role in fetal development particularly development of brain
- Role in skeletal development during childhood
- Inotropic (contractile) and chronotropic (rate) effects on the heart
- Regulation of bone marrow and mineralization.

Mechanism of Action

Thyroid hormones pass through the plasma membrane in their target cells to enter into cytosol where they can bind to specific proteins. This can maintain their concentration in the cytosol. Transport across the cell membrane is facilitated by well characterized cell membrane transporters. Mutations in genes transcribing these receptors lead to a situation simulating hypothyroidism but with high circulating thyroid hormone. Several classes of thyroid hormone transporters have been characterized. Their distribution and kinetics provides them with distinctive role in tissue specific thyroid hormone availability. Monocarboxylate transporter 8 is a specific thyroid hormone membrane transporter located on the X chromosome. Another transporter (Na^+ independent) organic anion transporting polypeptide is another well characterized transporter. There are different transporters for T4, T3, and rT3 except for brain where these hormones share same transporter.

True thyroid hormone receptors are chromosomally associated protein bound to response element of genomic DNA with associated repressor complex such as nuclear receptor corepressor (NCoR). The latter inhibits transcription. The binding of the thyroid hormone (ligand) to its receptor results in dissociation of repressor complex. This may be followed by addition of activator coregulators after which the gene is actively transcribed for the synthesis of numerous metabolic enzymes. High affinity thyroid hormone receptors are also present in inner mitochondrial membrane suggesting that thyroid hormones may directly regulate oxygen consumption and ATP production. Two genes (*THRA* and *THRB*) encode for two thyroid hormone receptors (TRα and TRβ). Each gene encodes for two major proteins generated by alternate splicing of mRNA. The *THRA* is expressed ubiquitously while *THRB* is restricted to liver, pituitary, retina, and few other areas of brain.

Regulation of Triiodothyronine and Thyroxine Synthesis

- Synthesis of T3 and T4 is controlled by feedback regulation
- Hormones T3 and T4 are more actively involved in regulatory process. Increased levels inhibit secretion of thyrotropin-releasing hormone (TRH) from hypothalamus and TSH from anterior pituitary
- On the contrary, decreased levels of T3 and T4 cause increased synthesis of TRH and TSH.

Evaluation of Thyroid Function

Basal metabolic rate (BMR) measurement was initially used for estimating thyroid gland activity. Later serum estimation of protein bound iodine was used to assess thyroid function. Now sensitive and reliable tests that include measurement of free or total T3, T4, and TSH by radioimmunoassay or enzyme-linked immunosorbent assay constitute the mainstay of laboratory evaluation. Normal concentration of these hormones is as follows:

- Free T3 = 1.7–4.2 pg/mL
- Free T4 = 0.7–1.80 ng/dL
- Total T3 = 80–200 ng/dL
- Total T4 = 5.0–12.4 µg/dL
- TSH = 0.35–5 mIU/mL.

Radioactive iodine uptake by the gland can localize thyroid gland and help in assessment of thyroid disorders.

THYROID-STIMULATING HORMONE LEVELS DURING PREGNANCY

- First trimester: 0.1–2.5 µIU/L
- Second trimester: 0.2–3.0 µIU/L
- Third trimester: 0.3–3.0 µIU/L

PATHOPHYSIOLOGY OF THYROID GLAND

Goiter: It is enlargement of thyroid gland. Thyroid-stimulating hormone level increases and thyroid gland enlarges in an attempt to compensate for decreased thyroid hormone production. Causes of this disease include:

- Iodide deficiency
- Iodide excess is less often associated with increase in thyroid mass
- Iodide transport defect
- Coupling defect
- Abnormal iodinated protein production
- Deficiency of deiodinase
- Iodination defect.

When the above described defects are severe, these lead to hypothyroidism and when these defects are partial, these lead to simple goiter. Goitrogenic substances are those that interfere with thyroid hormone production, e.g., nitrates, thiocyanates, perchlorates, etc.

Hypothyroidism: It can be consequent to defect in the pituitary, hypothalamus, or thyroid gland. It is caused due to deficiency of thyroid hormones and can occur in children (cretinism) or adults (myxedema). It can cause mental retardation in children but in adults, no mental retardation is observed. Symptoms include:
- Bradycardia (decreased heart rate)
- Lethargy and sleepiness
- Constipation
- Dry skin and hair
- Increased sensitivity to cold
- Hypothermia
- Worsening of kidney function and heart failure
- Anemia
- Excessive and prolonged menstrual bleeding in young females
- It is the most common endocrine cause of short stature in children.

Diagnosis is confirmed by elevated TSH in presence of low circulating thyroid hormone levels.

This disease can be treated by the exogenous supply of thyroid hormones.

Hyperthyroidism (thyrotoxicosis): It includes Graves' disease in which there is production of thyroid-stimulating IgG. The latter activates TSH receptor in thyroid gland due to which there is overproduction of thyroid hormones (T3 and T4).

Symptoms include:
- Tachycardia (increased heart rate)
- Nervousness

- Weight loss
- Weakness
- Moist skin
- Inability to sleep
- Protrusion of eye balls
- Tremors
- Excessive sweating.

Diagnosis is confirmed by documentation of low/suppressed TSH levels with concurrent high circulating levels of thyroid hormone(s).

Treatment includes use of antithyroid drug to block excessive production of thyroid hormones. In severe cases, thyroid gland may also be removed. In the United States, radioactive iodine use is the most preferred treatment modality.

Hashimoto's thyroiditis: It is an autoimmune disease (first to be recognized) in which thyroid gland becomes target of antibody mediated immune processes. This disease results in hypothyroidism with possible bouts of hyperthyroidism. The thyroid gland may enlarge not because of tissue hypertrophy but because of lymphocyte infiltration and fibrosis. There is gradual destruction of thyroid follicles due to antibodies against thyroid peroxidase and thyroglobulin. It is also known as chronic thyroiditis.

Symptoms include:
- Weight gain
- Chronic fatigue and muscle weakness
- Congestive heart failure
- Constipation
- Bradycardia (if hyperactive, tachycardia)
- Increased sensitivity to cold.

Diagnosis is confirmed by documentation of presence of thyroid peroxidase or antithyroglobulin antibodies. Treatment involves thyroid hormone replacement if circulating thyroid hormone levels are low.

Disease complex associated with thyroid hormone receptor dysfunction: A dysfunctional thyroid hormone receptor because of mutation in the gene transcribing the receptors leads to a situation of end-organ resistance. The cardinal feature of this state are elevated levels of free thyroxine and T3 levels with normal or slightly increased TSH concentration in absence of any major symptoms or signs of excess thyroid hormone. Depending upon which isoform of the receptor is dysfunctional, signs or symptoms vary.

Calcitonin

This hormone is discussed under the chapter "Hormones Regulating Calcium Metabolism".

APPLIED ASPECTS

- Thyroid hormone is a key metabolic regulator at all stages of life
- Thyroid gland is the exclusive site for thyroxine T4 production
- Triiodothyronine is dominantly derived from peripheral conversion of T4 to T3
- Thyroid hormones are bound to binding proteins (dominantly TBG) in circulation
- Triiodothyronine is the principal hormone for thyroid receptor having maximal avidity
- Thyroid hormones travel across plasma membrane via membrane transporters
- Inside the cell homodimerized or heterodimerized thyroid hormone receptors are attached to thyroid hormone response element of genomic DNA in conjunction with nuclear repressors (nCOR) that silences the gene transcription in basal state. When thyroid hormone binds to its designated site on the receptor (ligand binding domain),

the receptor complex sheds the nCOR and becomes a true transcription factor activating thyroid hormone responsive gene transcription downstream
- A set of symptoms and signs capture state of thyroid hormonal status—hypoactive or hyperactive state. Hormonal measurement helps define the syndromes
- Medical treatments are directed towards restoring free circulating thyroid hormone levels to desired targets (by oral replacement of thyroid hormone in hypothyroid states) or depleting levels of circulating hormones and restraining synthesis of new hormone in hyperthyroid states
- Acute illness impacts circulating thyroid hormones and might be confused with thyroid glandular dysfunction—a state referred to as nonthyroidal illness or previously designated as sick euthyroid state.

CHAPTER 6

Adrenal Gland

Adrenal glands are located above the kidneys are, therefore, called suprarenal glands. Each gland consists of an outer cortex and inner medulla. Each gland weighs approximately 4 grams. The cortex accounts for 90% of the mass with the remainder being medulla.

ADRENAL CORTEX

It produces around 50 steroid hormones (adrenocorticosteroids), but only some of these are biologically active. Adrenal cortex is differentiated into three regions:

- Zona glomerulosa: Outermost region producing mineralocorticoids (21-C) which regulate, water and electrolyte balance. The chief mineralocorticoid is aldosterone. Major stimulus is renin-angiotensin
- Zona fasciculata: It produces glucocorticoids (21-C) affecting glucose metabolism. Glucocorticoids also affect amino acid and fat metabolism. These actions are opposite to insulin. In humans, the most important glucocorticoid is cortisol and in rats, it is corticosterone. Major stimulus is adrenocorticotropic hormone (ACTH)
- Zona reticularis: Innermost region producing small quantities of androgens (19-C) and estrogens (18-C). Androgens and estrogens are mostly produced by the gonads. Dehydro-

epiandrosterone, a precursor to androgens and weak androgen, androstenedione are produced here. These are converted into more potent form in extra-adrenal tissue. Major stimulus is ACTH. Adrenocorticotropic hormone in turn depends on hypothalamic hormone—corticotropin releasing factor/hormone.

Biosynthesis of Adrenocorticosteroids

Cholesterol derived from plasma or synthesized in adrenal gland is the source for the synthesis of adrenocorticosteroids. After esterification, most of the cholesterol is stored in the cytoplasmic lipid droplets. Enzyme esterase is activated upon stimulation by ACTH and cholesterol formed from cholesteryl ester is transported into mitochondria where it is acted by cytochrome P-450 side chain cleavage enzyme to form pregnenolone (21-C) and isocaproaldehyde (Fig. 6.1). The reactions for the synthesis of adrenocorticosteroids take place in either mitochondria or endoplasmic reticulum (ER). In the first step of adrenal steroidogenesis, cholesterol enters mitochondria facilitated by steroidogenic acute regulatory protein. Five enzymes are involved in the synthesis of cortisol and six enzymes are involved in the synthesis of aldosterone.

Synthesis of mineralocorticoids: Enzymes 3β-hydroxysteroid dehydrogenase (3β-OHSD) and $\Delta^{5,4}$ isomerase act on pregnenolone and convert it into progesterone. The latter is acted upon by enzyme 21-hydroxylase forming 11-deoxycortisterone (a potent mineralocorticoid). Further hydroxylation by 11-hydroxylase leads to formation of corticosterone (weak mineralocorticoid). A mitochondrial enzyme 18-hydroxylase converts corticosterone into aldosterone with 18-hydroxycortisterone as an intermediate.

Synthesis of glucocorticoids: 17α-hydroxylase (SER enzyme and part of enzyme P450c17) acts on pregnenolone and pro-

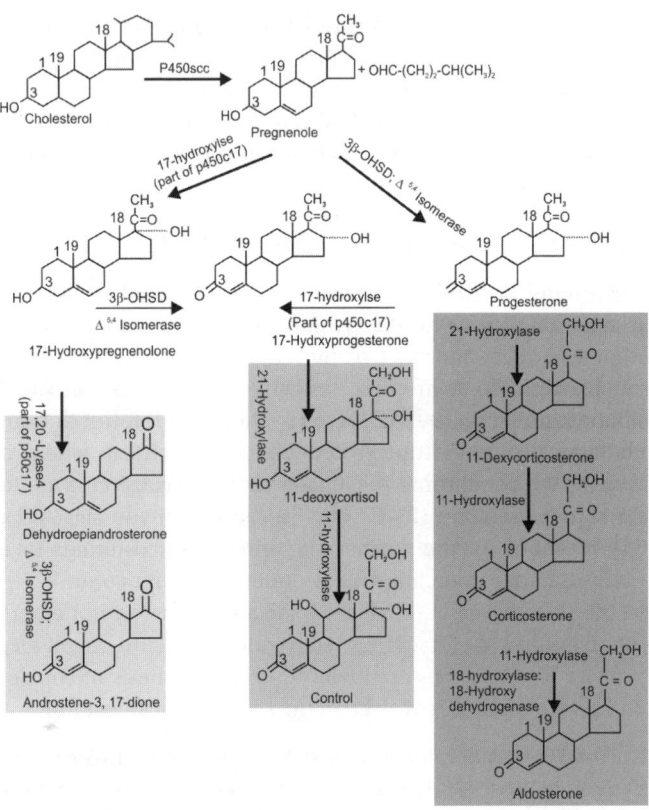

FIG. 6.1: Synthesis of adrenocorticoids

gesterone to produce 17-hydroxypregnenolone and 17-hydroxyprogesterone respectively. 17-hydroxypregnenolone can be converted to 17-hydroxyprogesterone in the presence of enzyme 3β-OHSD and $\Delta^{5,4}$ isomerase. 21-Hydroxylase (SER enzyme) converts 17-hydroxyprogesterone into 11-deoxycortisol which is later converted into cortisol (active glucocorticoid) by 11β-hydroxylase (mitochondrial enzyme), synthesis of glucocorticoids is dependent on stimulation by the ACTH secreted from anterior pituitary gland. Adrenocorticotropic hormone actions are rapid increasing adrenal glucocorticoid (cortisol) release into circulation within 30 minutes. Cortisol in turn has negative feedback control over ACTH secretion.

Synthesis of androgens: Small fraction of 17-hydroxypregnenolone undergoes oxidative fission by enzyme 17,20-lyase (part of enzyme P450c17) to produce weak androgen namely Dehydroepiandrosterone. The latter is converted into more potent androgen androstenedione by the combined action of enzyme 3β-OHSD and $\Delta^{5,4}$ isomerase. Enzyme 17,20-lyase can also act on 17-hydroxyprogesterone to form some amount of androstenedione. Some amount of testosterone can be produced from androstenedione by hydroxylation at C-17 position but most of this conversion takes place in the testes.

Adrenocorticosteroids—Biochemical Functions

Functions of Glucocorticoids

- They promote gluconeogenesis and thus increase blood glucose concentration. To promote gluconeogenesis, they increase gluconeogenic substrates particularly amino acids
- They increase circulating free fatty acids by promoting breakdown of stored triacylglycerol and reducing utilization of plasma free fatty acids
- At high concentration, they cause enhanced degradation of proteins in extrahepatic tissues (e.g., muscle, adipose tissue, etc.). In liver, they promote protein biosynthesis by stimulation of specific genes
- In high concentration, they suppress immune response by causing impairment of antibody synthesis or by damaging lymphocytes
- Deficiency of glucocorticoids causes increased production of ADH which may cause water retention in the body
- They inhibit bone formation and thus promote osteoporosis

- They may increase production of gastric hydrochloric acid and pepsinogen
- Increase cardiac contractility. Maintain vascular tone, and enhance vascular response to catecholamines
- Increase glomerular filtration rate and reduce calcium reabsorption
- Increase sodium retention and potassium excretion
- During fetal life stimulate production of surfactant by the fetal lung
- Maintain emotional balance and decrease rapid eye movement sleep.

Functions of Mineralocorticoids

- They promote reabsorption of Na^+ ions in the distal collecting tubule of the nephrons of the kidney. Retention of Na^+ ions is accomplished by corresponding excretion of K^+, H^+, and NH^{4+} ions.

Cellular Effects of Glucocorticoids

Many actions of glucocorticoids are mediated through classic glucocorticoid receptors that are ubiquitously expressed. Human glucocorticoid receptor (hGR) is the product of single gene located on chromosome 5. It contains 9 exons, and its alternate splicing results in two distinct mRNAs coding for hGRα and hGRβ. Each of these gene products produce additional isoforms depending on the site where translation of messenger RNA (mRNA) into protein is initiated. Glucocorticoid receptors undergo post-translation modification such as phosphorylation, ubiquitination, and sumoylation. The hGRα exists in the cytoplasm in association with heat shock protein (Hsp 90 and Hsp70). These are essential chaperons to induce conformational changes in the receptor allowing its ligand binding domain to receive and bind cortisol. Following this hGR dimerizes and translocates to nucleus binding to genomic glucocorticoid response element (GRE) to either stimulate or inhibit transcription of glucocorticoid responsive genes. Alternatively it may bind to other transcription factors such as STAT or NFkB to stimulate or inhibit their transcriptional activity. Unlike the hGRα, hGRβ is contained within the nucleus of the cell and does not bind to GRE and therefore, remains transcriptionally inactive. It has been shown to be a dominant inhibitor of the transcriptional activity of hGRα and may thus determine tissue specific sensitivity to glucocorticoids.

Although most of the glucocorticoid activity is mediated by nuclear receptors, there is considerable evidence that some effects might be mediated by cell membrane or cytoplasmic receptors. One of the most notable nongenomic actions is the rapid phosphorylation of annexin-1 that inhibits activation of phospholipase (PL) A2 via the EGF receptor. Other nongenomic effects include activation of PI3 kinase inhibition of voltage gated calcium channels and stimulation of GABA release.

In circulation cortisol is transported bound to high affinity corticosteroid binding globulin (CBG or transcortin). Normally, it carries approximately 90% of the circulating hormone. A smaller fraction 6–10% is bound to low affinity but high capacity protein—albumin. Less than 5% is unbound or free. Cortisol has a half-life of 70–120 minutes and it is primarily metabolized in the liver.

At the pre-receptor level, glucocorticoid activity is regulated by 11β-hydroxysteroid dehydrogenase. It has two isoforms: 11β-HSD1 and 11β-HSD 2. Former is a bidirectional enzyme that converts cortisone to cortisol and back. Latter is unidirectional dehydrogenase that converts cortisol into inactive cortisone. While 11β-HSD1 is widely distributed, 11β-HSD2 exhibits a narrow and distinct tissue restricted expression (such as distal tubule of kidney, colon, and salivary gland). This prevents cortisol from interacting with mineralocorticoid receptor for which it has equal affinity. This enzyme thus serves as a gate keeper for cortisol exposure to its receptor.

Cellular Effects of Mineralocorticoids

Aldosterone circulates bound to its binding protein. Unbound (free) aldosterone diffuses across the cell membrane in the kidney, colon, and salivary glands. Its actions in kidneys have been well studied. Once it crosses the cell membrane, it interacts with its receptor (mineralocorticoid receptor-MR). Once activated these receptors dimerize and then translocate to nucleus where they induce transcription of serum glucocorticoid-activated kinase. This enhances expression of the epithelial Na^+ channel and Na^+/K^+ ATPase transporters thereby increasing sodium and water reabsorption. Activated mineralocorticoid receptors may induce expression/trafficking of these channels by non-genomic mechanisms too as is the expression of H^+- ATPase pumps in the apical membrane.

Control of aldosterone synthesis and release operates through renin-angiotensin system. Renin response is finely calibrated by the intravascular volume.

PATHOPHYSIOLOGY OF ADRENAL CORTEX

Glucocorticoids Related Disorders

Adrenal insufficiency: It is caused by failure of adrenal gland to secrete glucocorticoids. Overall, the most important cause is the sudden withdrawal of exogenous glucocorticoids. Adrenal insufficiency may be primary or secondary.

Primary adrenal insufficiency is also known as Addison's disease. This diagnosis assumes that primary glucocorticoid secretory abnormality rests with the adrenal gland while functions of pituitary and hypothalamus are intact. One would therefore see low circulating plasma cortisol levels with consequent elevated levels of ACTH, and CRH (not generally measured). Other causes include destruction of adrenal gland by overwhelming infection, metastases from malignant tumors (most commonly lungs) or autoimmunity; bleeding inside the gland; drugs interfering with glucocorticoids metabolism; or impaired synthesis of glucocorticoids due to deficiency of enzyme(s) involved in steroid biosynthesis.

Symptoms include:
- Hypoglycemia
- Loss in weight
- Weakness
- Anorexia (loss of appetite)
- Nausea
- Hypotension (low blood pressure)
- Decreased plasma Na^+ levels
- Increased plasma K^+ levels
- Increased lymphocyte and eosinophil counts
- Hyperpigmentation of skin. It is the hallmark of primary adrenal insufficiency.

Secondary adrenal insufficiency: It is caused due to deficiency of ACTH due to infection, tumor, or infarction involving pituitary gland. It may be caused by isolated ACTH deficiency or sometime seen after inflammation of pituitary (hypophysitis). Often it is seen following prolonged use of exogenous steroids. Symptoms are similar as above but there is no hyperpigmentation or dominance of electrolyte imbalance. In secondary adrenal insufficiency ACTH levels are also low/suppressed.

Cushing syndrome: It is caused due to excess of glucocorticoids which may be due to steroid use, pituitary adenoma (releasing excessive ACTH) ,adrenal adenoma, or ectopic production of ACTH by tumors outside the pituitary (lung, pancreas). Symptoms include:
- Hyperglycemia or glucose intolerance
- Muscle wasting

- Osteoporosis
- Hypertension
- Truncal obesity and fullness of supraclavicular fat pads
- Decreased resistance to infections and inflammatory response.

Mineralocorticoids-associated Disorders

Conn's syndrome (primary aldosteronism): It is caused due to excessive aldosterone production due to adenomas in zona glomerulosa. Symptoms include:
- Increased blood Na^+ (hypernatremia)
- Decreased blood K^+ (hypokalemia)
- Hypertension
- Alkalosis
- Suppression of plasma renin levels.

In most cases, the disease arises due to single adrenal cortical adenoma secreting aldosterone autonomously (unilateral disease) or bilateral adrenal hyperplasia. Unilateral disease is cured by surgical resection while bilateral disease is not amenable to surgery. Because of sodium retention and intravascular volume expansion, plasma renin levels are often suppressed. Other causes of hyperaldosteronism include, unilateral adrenal hyperplasia, glucocorticoid remediable aldosteronism, and adrenal carcinoma.

Glucocorticoid remediable aldosteronism is an autosomal dominant disorder and is also known as familial hyperaldosteronism type I. In this condition, promoter sequence of 11β-hydroxylase gene is fused with aldosterone synthase gene making aldosterone synthase dependent on ACTH. Hence it becomes "glucocorticoid remediable" since exogenous glucocorticoid would suppress ACTH and thereby aldosterone synthase activation.

Secondary aldosteronism: It is caused due to hyperfunction and hyperplasia of juxtaglomerular cells which results in elevated levels of renin and consequent formation of angiotensin II. Symptoms are almost similar as for primary aldosteronism. It is often seen as a result of intravascular volume depletion from overzealous use of diuretics (water pills) to treat hypertension, or congestive heart failure. Renin levels are always elevated in this situation.

An important medical entity for which screening at birth is mandated pertains to inborn errors of steroid hormone biosynthesis. Untreated it poses serious threat to life. The nature of disease depends upon which biosynthetic enzyme is absent or insufficient. The most common deficiency encountered in clinical practice is 21-hydroxylase deficiency. This results in cortisol and aldosterone and therefore severe dehydration and marked elevation in serum potassium.

ADRENAL MEDULLA

Adrenal medulla is an extension of sympathetic nervous system. Chromaffin cells in adrenal medulla produce catecholamines namely epinephrine, norepinephrine, and dopamine. Both norepinephrine and dopamine act as neurotransmitters in brain and autonomic nervous system. Sympathetic ganglion cells are also present in the gland. Chromaffin cells are so named because of characteristic staining with chromic acid.

Biosynthesis of Catecholamines

Catecholamines are synthesized from amino acid tyrosine in the chromaffin cells of the adrenal medulla. About 80% of formed catecholamine in adrenal medulla is epinephrine and none of it is made in the extramedullary tissue whereas most of the norepinephrine is made in the organs innervated by sympathetic nervous system or in the nerve endings. Formation of epinephrine from tyrosine involves four major steps:

1. Tyrosine hydroxylase (rate limiting enzyme) converts tyrosine into dihydroxyphenylalanine (Levodopa). This enzyme acts as an oxidoreductase and uses tetrahydropteridine as a cofactor
2. Dopa decarboxylase converts Levodopa into dopamine (3, 4-dihydroxyphenylethylamine). This enzyme requires pyridoxal phosphate as the cofactor. Levodopa can be used in the treatment of Parkinson's disease (caused by local deficiency of dopamine in brain) as it can easily cross blood brain barrier
3. Dopamine β-hydroxylase converts dopamine into norepinephrine. This enzyme is rich in secretory granules of medullary cells and uses fumarate as a modulator
4. Phenylethanolamine-N-Methyltransferase causes N-methylation of norepinephrine to form epinephrine. Phenylethanolamine-N-Methyltransferase is induced by glucocorticoid hormone (Fig. 6.2).

Catecholamines are stored in secretory granules in association with adenosine triphosphate (ATP) and a number of other proteins including adrenomedullin. The output of catecholamines is controlled by nerve cells within posterior hypothalamus. The signal travels down via spinal cord ultimately stimulating cholinergic pre-ganglion nerve fibers innervating adrenal medulla. The half-life of catecholamines in circulation is very short (1–2 minutes).

Mechanism of Action of Epinephrine

Catecholamine action is triggered by binding of catecholamines to G-protein linked to membrane receptor. On

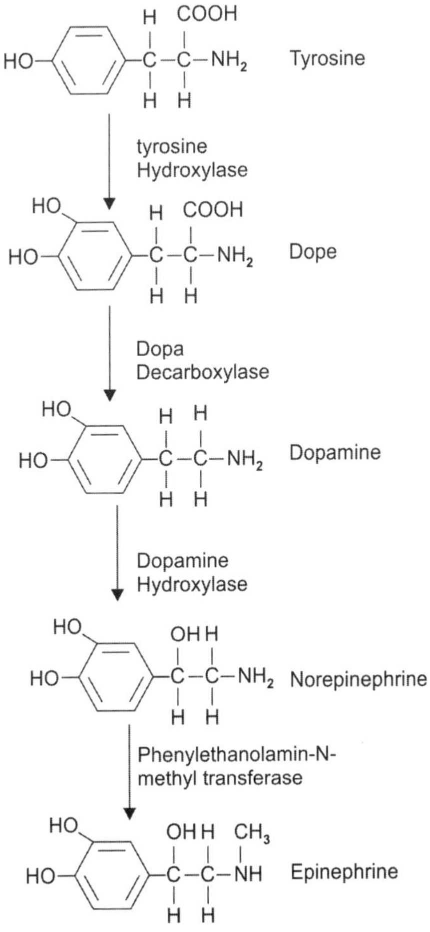

FIG. 6.2: Synthesis of catecholamines in adrenal medulla

activation, there is increased production of cyclic adenosine monophosphate. These receptors are classified α- or β-adrenergic receptors based on their physiological or pharmacological effects induced up on hormone binding, Epinephrine bound to adrenergic receptors on the surface of heart muscle cell increases contraction rate resulting in increased blood supply to the tissues. In contrast, stimulation of β-adrenergic of the intestine causes their relaxation. Epinephrine also stimulates α_2 adrenergic receptors found on smooth muscle cell lining of the blood vessels in the intestinal tract, skin, and kidneys, causes the arteries to constrict and thus reducing their blood supply. These different effects of epinephrine have a common result, i.e., supplying energy for the rapid movement of major locomotor muscles in response to stress such as fright or heavy exercise.

Catecholamines' Biochemical Functions

- Both epinephrine and norepinephrine enhance lipolysis in adipose tissue which increases the concentration of free fatty acids in the circulation. Increased fatty acids are used as a source of energy for heart and muscle
- Catecholamines particularly epinephrine increase cardiac output and blood pressure. They cause smooth muscle contraction of blood vessels supplying skin and kidney while smooth muscle relaxation of blood vessels supplying skeletal muscle
- Miscellaneous: Dilation of pupils, contraction of spleen, and inhibition of micturition (urination).

PATHOPHYSIOLOGY OF ADRENAL MEDULLA

Pheochromocytoma: It is a tumor of adrenal medulla associated with excessive production of epinephrine and norepinephrine. It is often associated with sustained or periodic severe hypertension. Symptoms include palpitation, profuse sweating, and headaches. This triad of symptoms is quite impressive. Patients experience spells of this triad and describe a sense of doom. Pheochromocytomas are uncommon per se, and arise from intra-adrenal chromaffin tissue as mentioned above. When catecholamine secreting tumors arise outside the adrenal gland (extra-adrenal) they are called paragangliomas. These tumors may be sporadic or may be genetically inherited. Several candidate genes have been identified and syndromes well described. These include:

- The von Hippel-Lindau (*VHL*) gene
- RET gene associated with multiple endocrine neoplasia 2 (*MEN2*)
- Neurofibromatosis type 1 gene (*NF1*)
- Genes encoding B, C, and D subunits of succinate dehydrogenase
- Gene encoding succinate dehydrogenase 5.

Surgical removal is the treatment of choice. Measurement of plasma free metanephrines is 100% sensitive for diagnosis. Pending surgery control of hypertension by α receptor blockers such as phenoxybenzamine is very important. Physicians have considerable experience using these agents.

CHAPTER 7

Hormones Regulating Calcium Metabolism

Calcium is an important element that plays key role in many systems and cellular processes. In human body, there is about 1.2 kg of calcium of which 99% resides in skeleton and teeth. In bones, calcium occurs with phosphate in the form of hydroxyapatite crystals. Most of the calcium is not exchanged with extracellular fluid but some amount (approximately 1%) can exchange with extracellular fluid. Hormones parathormone [parathyroid hormone (PTH)] secreted by parathyroid gland and calcitriol secreted by kidneys, influence mobilization of calcium to make it available for cellular activities. Most of the intracellular calcium is sequestered in the endoplasmic reticulum, mitochondria, and sarcoplasmic reticulum (muscle) with very small amount of free calcium approximately 0.1 µmol/L. Control of calcium and phosphate are intimately connected and this appreciation goes long way in understanding metabolic/mineral disorders. Most of body's phosphate (95%) is also in skeleton.

Plasma calcium is found to exist in mainly three forms:
- Protein bound Calcium: Calcium is bound to proteins like albumin. Protein binding prevents ectopic calcification as calcium along with phosphorous occurs near the solubility product in the plasma. Deficiency of albumin can result in

decrease of plasma total calcium level. Alkalosis increases calcium binding with proteins and thus decreases the concentration of ionized calcium
- Calcium complexed with organic acids: Calcium in plasma may be bound to citric acid, phosphoric acid, etc.
- Ionized Calcium: It is the biologically active form of calcium. It represents 45% of extracellular calcium.

It is important to maintain normal level of ionized calcium as it plays a major role in the following biochemical functions:
- Muscle contraction
- Blood coagulation
- Hormone secretion
- Intracellular second messenger for several hormones
- Activation of protein kinase C
- Neuromuscular excitability
- Plasma membrane transport
- Membrane integrity
- Enzyme reactions
- Bone mineralization.

Phosphate has multiple important functions as well such as:
- Formation of high energy compounds such as adenosine triphosphate, creatine phosphate
- Formation of active signaling molecules
- Important intracellular ion
- Major component of deoxyribonucleic acid/ribonucleic acid (DNA/RNA) and membrane phospholipids
- Role in bone mineralization.

Hormones regulating calcium homeostasis include:
- Parathyroid hormone (produced in parathyroid gland)
- Calcitriol (produced in kidney)
- Calcitonin (produced in thyroid gland).

PARATHYROID HORMONE

There are two pairs of parathyroid glands associated with bilobed thyroid gland. The chief cells of the parathyroid gland synthesize PTH. The latter acts on three organs namely bone, kidney, and intestine to maintain total calcium in the range of 8.5–10.5 mg/dL. The ionized fraction controls the secretion of PTH. The PTH secretion increases at low calcium and decreases at high calcium.

Biosynthesis of Parathyroid Hormone

Parathyroid hormone is made of 84 amino acids and is formed from proparathyroid hormone (ProPTH) (90 amino acid). Proparathyroid hormone has highly basic hexapeptide amino terminal extension. Proparathyroid hormone is made from 115 amino acid pre-ProPTH which has additional 25 amino acid hydrophobic amino terminal extension. Parathyroid hormone (1-34) has full biological activity and the region PTH (18-34) is required for binding to the receptor on the target cells. Residues 1-6 are required for receptor activation (Fig. 7.1).

Most of the ProPTH synthesized in the parathyroid cell is degraded and it is found that the rate of this degradation

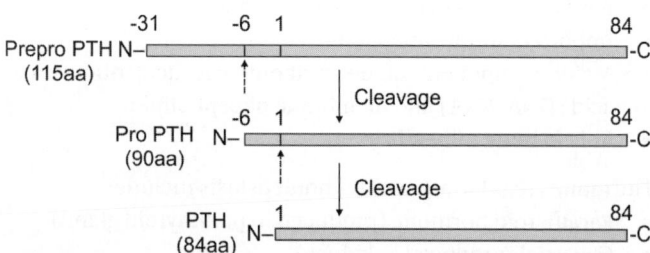

FIG. 7.1: Formation of parathyroid hormone from preproparathormone

decreases when Ca^{2+} levels are low and increases when Ca^{2+} levels are high. These effects are mediated by the Ca^{2+} receptor on the surface of parathyroid cells. Proteolytic enzymes cleaving pre-ProPTH, ProPTH, and PTH have been located in parathyroid tissue. Cathepsin B cleaves PTH into PTH_{1-36} (can be rapidly cleaved into di- and tripeptides) and PTH_{37-84} (not degraded further). After secretion, PTH can also undergo proteolytic cleavage in other tissues like liver.

The control of PTH secretion is exerted through unique G-protein coupled calcium sensing receptor (CaSR). When ionized calcium levels rise above 1.2 mmols/L, CaSR is activated and PTH secretion inhibited. Calcium sensing receptor is found on both chief cells (where it inhibits PTH expression, synthesis, and release) and C-cells where it stimulates secretion of calcitonin. High levels of calcitriol also inhibit PTH synthesis.

Parathyroid Hormone-biochemical Functions

- Parathyroid hormone stimulates osteoclasts to cause demineralization of bone. This leads to loss of calcium from the bones which increase calcium levels in the blood. To cause bone demineralization, PTH causes increased activity of enzymes pyrophosphatase and collagenase
- Parathyroid hormone increases reabsorption of calcium from the nephrons of the kidneys to increase blood calcium levels
- Parathyroid hormone promotes the synthesis of calcitriol (by stimulation of 1α hydroxylase enzyme in kidneys) which increases intestinal absorption of calcium to elevate blood calcium levels
- Parathyroid hormone decreases blood phosphate levels by increasing renal phosphate clearance.

Parathyroid hormone has two G-protein coupled receptors (PTH-1 receptor and PTH-2 receptor) designated as PTHR1 and PTHR2. Parathyroid hormone and its related hormone PTH-related peptide can act via PTHR1, but only PTH acts on PTHR2. Receptor stimulation results in activation of adenylate cyclase/cyclic adenosine monophosphate (cAMP) pathway.

Pathophysiology of Parathyroid Gland

Hypoparathyrodism: Parathyroid hormone levels are low due to autoimmune destruction of parathyroid gland (primary hypoparathyrodism) or due to damage to the gland during neck surgery (secondary hypoparathyrodism). Alternatively, it may be consequence of developmental abnormality or infiltrative disorders. Antibodies directed against CaSR have been identified in patients with autoimmune hypoparathyrodism. These antibodies possibly result in functional activation of receptor leading to inhibition of PTH secretion. A combination of low calcium and PTH may be seen in situations where Magnesium levels are concurrently low.

In this condition, there is decreased serum calcium and increased serum phosphate levels. Symptoms include:
- Mild hypocalcemia causes muscle cramps and tetany
- Severe hypocalcemia causes tetanic paralysis of respiratory muscles
- Chronic hypocalcemia can cause cataract or cutaneous changes
- Congestive heart failure.

Pseudohypoparathyroidism: In this condition, there is end organ resistance to effects of PTH. It results from mutations in *GNAS1* gene encoding alpha subunit of G-protein coupled to PTH receptor Symptoms are same as described above. In addition, patient can suffer from mental retardation and developmental abnormalities. As against hypoparathyroidism, the circulating levels of PTH are elevated. It is further subdivided in two groups depending on presence or absence of classical phenotypic abnormalities. The expression of *GNAS1* gene follows imprinting where expression of the allele in a tissue depends on whether the allele is maternally inherited or paternally inherited.

Hyperparathyroidism: Parathyroid hormone levels are high due to parathyroid adenoma (85% cases) or parathyroid hyperplasia. Serum calcium levels are high and serum phosphate levels are low. It is most frequent cause of hypercalcemia in nonhospitalized patients. It usually appears in fifth to sixth decade of life and may be totally asymptomatic as long as person remains well hydrated. An earlier presentation should evoke consideration of a familial cause such as multiple endocrine neoplasia 1 and less commonly MEN2. A rare, but important condition is hyperparathyroidism jaw tumor syndrome. Carcinoma of parathyroid gland is common in this condition. It is often associated with mutation of gene *HRPT2* which encodes a protein called parafibromin.

Symptoms and laboratory abnormalities include:
- Increased resorption of bones causing increased susceptibility to fractures
- Decreased renal function, kidney stones, and urinary tract infections
- High plasma calcitriol
- Low plasma bicarbonate
- Fatigue
- Failure to concentrate
- Increased thirst
- Abdominal pains from renal colic.

CALCITRIOL

Vitamin D (a fat soluble vitamin) is steroid in nature and functions like a hormone. Major source of endogenous vitamin D (cholecalciferol) is skin where 7-dehydrocholesterol (formed in the course of cholesterol biosynthesis) is converted into cholecalciferol (vitamin D3) on exposure to sunlight (ultraviolet B). Vitamin D3 is not biologically active. From skin, it is transported to liver bound to vitamin D binding protein. It is metabolized in the body through two hydroxylations to form biologically active form.

Biosynthesis of Calcitriol

Calcitriol is produced in the kidneys but its precursors are produced in the skin and liver. The steps include:
- Cholecalciferol is produced in the skin from 7-dehydrocholesterol on exposure to sunlight (ultraviolet B)
- Cholecalciferol is then hydroxylated at 25th position to produce 25-hydroxycholecalciferol (25-OH D3). This reaction takes place in the liver by a specific hydroxylase namely calciol 25-hydroxylase. The latter requires cytochrome P450, NADPH, and molecular oxygen for the hydroxylation process. The 25-OH D3 is the major circulatory form of vitamin D and is also called calcidiol
- Enzyme 1α-hydroxylase converts calcidiol into calcitriol (1,25-dihydroxycholecalciferol). Calcitriol has 3 OH groups at position 1, 3, and 25. Enzyme 1α-hydroxylase requires cytochrome P450, NADPH and molecular oxygen for the hydroxylation process.

Regulation of Calcitriol synthesis

Plasma calcium and phosphate levels regulate production of calcitriol in the kidneys. Low Ca^{2+} levels promote the production of PTH which activates enzyme 1α-Hydroxylase. Low plasma PO_4^{2-} on the other hand directly increases the activity of enzyme 1α-hydroxylase. On the other hand, this enzyme is inhibited by *FGF23* (Fig. 7.2).

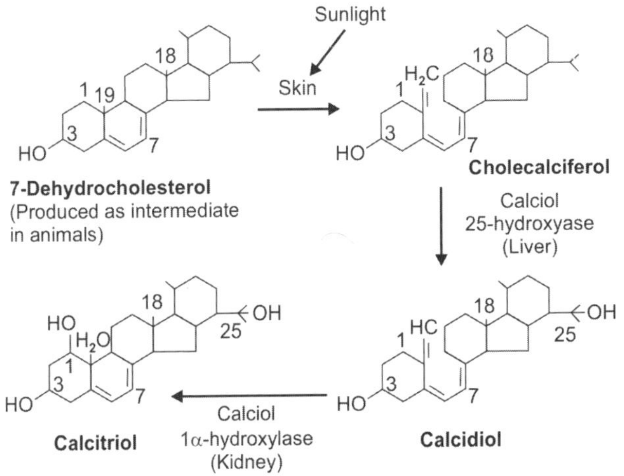

FIG. 7.2: Biosynthesis of calcitriol

Calcitriol-biochemical Functions

Calcitriol acts on three organs, namely, intestine, kidney, and bone to maintain the plasma calcium levels. Calcitriol increases the blood calcium levels.

1. Action on intestine: Being steroid in nature, calcitriol enters the plasma membrane of intestinal cells and combine with cytosolic receptor. Hormone receptor complex so formed migrates into the nucleus and interacts with specific DNA sites leading to the synthesis of specific calcium binding protein. The latter increases the intake of calcium from the intestinal lumen into the blood
2. Action on bone: Calcitriol is essential for bone formation as it stimulates the uptake of calcium for its deposition as calcium phosphate in the bones. Calcitriol also increases the mobilization of calcium and phosphate from the bones to elevate plasma calcium levels
3. Action on kidney: It decreases the excretion of calcium and phosphate from the kidneys so that more calcium is retained in the plasma.

Justification for Vitamin D acting as a Hormone

Following points justify the status of vitamin D as a hormone:
- Calcitriol, the biologically active form of vitamin D is produced in the kidney
- The action of calcitriol is similar to the action of a steroid hormone
- Calcitriol like other hormones acts on target organs, namely, intestine, bone, and kidney
- Calcitriol is synthesized in the body cells, i.e. kidney
- Calcitriol synthesis is self-regulated.

Disorders Associated with Vitamin D Deficiency and Excess

Hypovitaminosis D: It is caused by insufficient exposure to sunlight, strict vegetarian diet, disorder in liver and kidney, or fat malabsorption syndrome. This causes rickets in children and osteomalacia in adults. Symptoms include:
- Soft and pliable bones
- Delay in teeth formation
- Increase in alkaline phosphatase activity due to increased cell activity in the bone
- Soft bones increasing their susceptibility to fractures.

Renal rickets: These are caused by decreased synthesis of calcitriol due to chronic renal failure. This decreases the calcium levels in the blood.

Hypervitaminosis D: Vitamin D is stored in the liver and slowly metabolized. It is the most toxic vitamin in overdosed state. There is increased level of calcium in the blood. Symptoms include:
- Increased resorption of bone
- Deposition of calcium in soft tissues such as kidney and arteries
- Kidney stones

- Loss of appetite
- Increased thirst giving way to reduced thirst
- Weight loss.

Levels of 25-OH Vitamin D_3

- Deficiency: <20 ng/mL
- Insufficiency: 20–30 ng/mL
- Sufficiency: 30–100 ng/mL
- Toxicity: >100 ng/mL.

CALCITONIN

Parafollicular C-cells of thyroid are the source of this hormone. C-cells originate in the neural crest and are related to the cells of other endocrine glands. It is released in response to hypercalcemia and gastrin. It is an important biomarker for C-cell hyperplasia and medullary thyroid carcinoma.

- Calcitonin is formed by proteolytic cleavage of pre-propeptide (product of *CALC1* gene). Alternative splicing of this gene can also produce distantly related peptide called calcitonin gene-related peptide
- Calcitonin is a 32 amino acid peptide hormone
- Calcitonin has a 7 member N-terminal loop formed by Cys-Cys bridge. This loop is required for the biological activity of calcitonin
- Receptor for calcitonin is present in osteoclasts, kidney, and regions of brain. Its receptor is a G protein-coupled receptor which is coupled to enzyme adenylate cyclase by G_s. Thus, its actions are due to increased levels of cAMP.

Calcitonin-biochemical Functions

Calcitonin lowers the blood calcium levels and thus works antagonistic to PTH. Its function is not significant in the regulation of calcium homeostasis. To lower blood calcium levels:

- It inhibits osteoclastic resorption of bone by stimulating cAMP synthesis in osteoclasts. During periods of calcium mobilization (as in pregnancy and lactation), calcitonin protects against calcium loss from the skeleton. Parathyroid hormone also increases cAMP levels, but how the action of calcitonin and PTH are different is still unclear
- It inhibits calcium reabsorption from kidneys by acting on cells different from those which are stimulated by PTH
- It inhibits calcium reabsorption from the intestine
- Calcitonin has been used to treat patients presenting with acute hypercalcemia. Its effects however wane rapidly (tachyphylaxis) hence it is not suited for long-term therapy. A basal preparation has been used to treat osteoporosis.

CHAPTER 8

Pancreas

Pancreas is a heterocrine gland acting both as exocrine gland (acinar lobules) and endocrine gland (islet of Langerhans). Islet of Langerhans has four different types of cells; namely; (i) α cells (secreting glucagon), (ii) β cells (secreting insulin), (iii) δ cells (secreting somatostatin), and (iv) F cells or PP cells (secreting pancreatic polypeptide). Its primary endocrine function is to secrete insulin and glucagon to control metabolism of circulating fuels. Its exocrine function pertains to release of enzymes involved in digestion process and also providing bicarbonate rich fluid to allow enzyme digest/process ingested food.

INSULIN

It is a polypeptide hormone having major influence on carbohydrate, protein, and fat metabolism. As it promotes synthesis of proteins, triglycerides, and glycogen, it is called anabolic hormone. Insulin was the first hormone to be synthesized, purified, and sequenced and the first hormone to be made by recombinant DNA technology. The first hormone to have been isolated and synthesized was the adrenal hormone epinephrine (identified by Jokichi Takamine in 1901).

Insulin Structure

It is made up of two polypeptide chains A and B. A chain has 21 amino acids and B chain has 30 amino acids. There are two interchain disulphide bonds (connecting A_7 to B_7 and A_{20} to B_{19}) and one intrachain disulphide bond (connecting A_6 to A_{11}). Most of the mammalian insulins have same molecular weight of 5808 Da. However, no two mammalian insulins are identical in structure. Porcine insulin is closest to human insulin. It differs from human insulin by one amino acid whereas bovine insulin is different by three amino acids. Previously when recombinant insulin was not available, these two insulins were used for the treatment of insulin requiring diabetic patients. Guinea pig insulin is different by 17 amino acids from human insulin, and therefore, guinea pig is the animal in which antibodies to human insulin are raised for radioimmunoassay or enzyme-linked immunosorbent assay assays. Biological activity of most mammalian insulins is similar, i.e., 25 units/mg protein. Human synthesizes roughly 2 mg insulin daily.

Insulin Biosynthesis

The gene for insulin synthesis is located on chromosome 11. Insulin is produced from proinsulin which is formed from pre-proinsulin. Preproinsulin (108 amino acids) is converted to proinsulin (86 amino acids) in endoplasmic reticulum and signal sequence is liberated. The structure of proinsulin is shown in figure 8.1. Proinsulin is sequentially degraded in golgi apparatus to form active hormone insulin and C-peptide in equimolar concentration. The estimation of C-peptide in the plasma serves as a useful index to know about endogenous production of insulin. Insulin and proinsulin form complexes with zinc and in this form it is stored in cytoplasmic granules of β cells. How insulin is synthesized was uncovered by Don Steiner and his group at the University of Chicago.

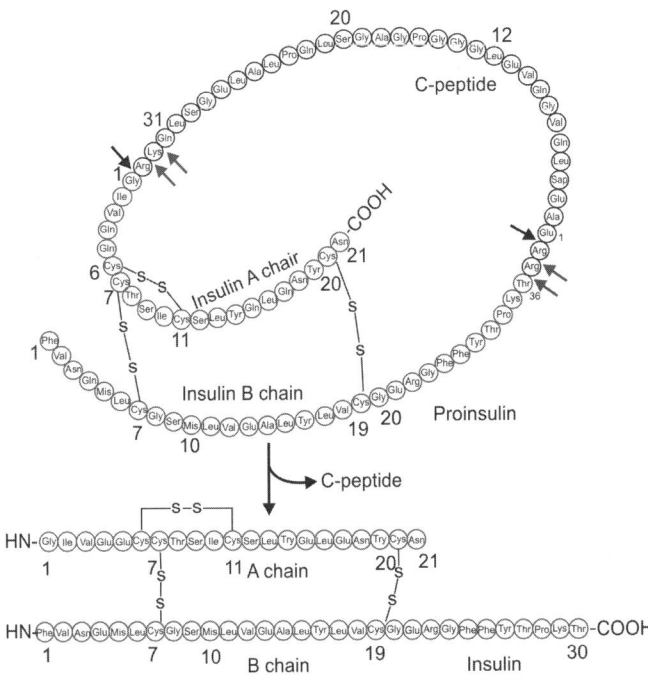

FIG. 8.1: Biosynthesis of insulin from proinsulin. Note the presence of brown colored C-peptide in structure of proinsulin. Cleavage sites are shown by arrows. Carboxypeptidase-like enzyme (gray arrow) and trypsin-like enzyme (black arrow) cleave proinsulin to form insulin

Insulin Secretion and Its Regulation

Factors Promoting Insulin Release

- Glucose: Administration of glucose or carbohydrates (which yield glucose on digestion) through diet is the key signal for insulin secretion. Glucose enters the pancreatic β cells of the islets through glucose transporter 2 (GLUT2) to equilibrate glucose concentration across the cell

membrane. As the cellular concentration of glucose rises, it increases the conversion of glucose to glucose-6-phosphate by glucokinase. As a consequence the increase in metabolism of glucose-6-phosphate in the mitochondria generates adenosine triphosphate (ATP) and tilts ratio in favor of ATP:ADP (adenosine diphosphate). It is followed by the closure of ATP-sensitive potassium channels causing membrane depolarization of the β cells which leads to opening of voltage-sensitive calcium channels, a rise in intracellular calcium triggering release of insulin. Insulin secretion from the β cells occurs in two distinct phase: (i) first phase of insulin release (FPIR) occurring with 5 minutes of β cell exposure to glucose, and (ii) a second phase which occurs later
- Amino acids: Rise in plasma amino acids after a protein rich meal induces the secretion of insulin. Amino acids arginine and lysine are most effective in promoting insulin release
- Gastrointestinal hormones: Gastrointestinal hormones released after ingestion of food, namely, secretin, gastrin, glucagon-like peptide 1 and 2 (GLP-1 and GLP-2), and glucose-dependent insulinotropic polypeptide (GIP; previously known as gastric-inhibitory polypeptide) promote secretion of insulin. The GIP is now named as glucose-dependent insulinotropic polypeptide. Glucose-dependent insulinotropic polypeptide is released from the K-cells located near duodenum and upper jejunum while GLP-1 and GLP-2 are secreted by the L-endocrine cells located in distal ileum and colon
- Ketone bodies.

Factors Inhibiting Insulin Release

- Epinephrine: It is released during stress from adrenal medulla and is most potent inhibitor of release of insulin.

In emergency situation, epinephrine provides fuels in circulation by releasing fatty acids from adipose tissue and glucose from liver
- Somatostatin released by the D-cells is a potent inhibitor of insulin as well as glucagon.

Insulin Degradation

The normal concentration of fasting plasma insulin is 2–25 µIU/mL. Plasma insulin has a short half-life of around 5 minutes. Most of the insulin is degraded in liver and some in kidneys. The insulin degrading enzyme is generically referred to as insulinase. About 50% of hepatic portal insulin is cleared through the liver during its first pass. The kidney is the major site for insulin clearance from the systemic circulation. In conditions where kidney functions are failing or have failed, the half-life of circulating insulin is prolonged.

Insulin-biochemical Functions

Effect on Carbohydrate Metabolism

- Insulin promotes utilization and storage of glucose. It causes glucose uptake in muscles, adipose tissue, white blood cells, etc. and also promotes glucose utilization in liver but glucose entry into liver may not be dependent on insulin
- Insulin increases glycolysis in muscle and liver by activating regulatory enzymes namely glucokinase, phosphofructokinase, and pyruvate kinase
- Insulin increases activity of glycogen synthase (increasing glycogenesis) and decreases activity of glycogen phosphorylase (decreasing glycogenolysis)
- Insulin also suppresses gluconeogenesis by decreasing the activity of enzymes phosphoenolpyruvate carboxykinase and glucose-6-phosphatase.

Effect on Lipid Metabolism

- Adipose tissue is most sensitive to action of insulin. Insulin promotes lipogenesis by promoting triglyceride synthesis from glycerol-3-phosphate (derived from glycolysis) and nicotinamide adenine dinucleotide phosphate (from hexose monophosphate shunt)
- Insulin promotes fatty acid synthesis by activating key enzyme acetyl-CoA carboxylase. The activity of hormone-sensitive lipase is decreased by insulin which lowers the breakdown of stored fat in the adipose tissue
- Insulin decreases ketogenesis by promoting the activity of hydroxymethylglutaryl CoA synthase and increasing utilization of acetyl CoA.

Effect on Protein Metabolism

- Insulin promotes protein synthesis and reduces protein degradation. For protein synthesis, it stimulates amino acids entry into the cells.

Other Functions

- With the help from epidermal growth factor platelet-derived growth factor, and prostaglandins, insulin promotes cell growth and replication (Fig. 8.2).

Mechanism of Insulin Action or Signal Transduction

- Insulin receptor mediated signal transduction: Insulin receptor is heterodimer containing 2α chains and 2β chains ($\alpha_2\beta_2$) (Fig. 8.2). Both the subunits are held together by disulphide bonds. The α-subunit contains site for binding to insulin and is present extracellularly. The β-subunit is a transmembrane protein and has tyrosine kinase activity on its cytoplasmic domain. The α-subunit regulates the tyrosine kinase activity of the intracellular domain of the β-subunit

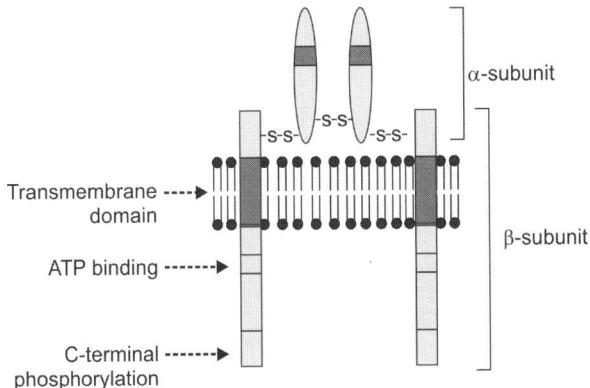

ATP, adenosine triphosphate.

FIG. 8.2: Insulin receptor

- The insulin receptor has a short half-life of 6–12 hours. The number of these receptors per cell is very high (about 20,000 per cell). Binding of insulin to the α-subunit induces conformational change in it and this signal is transduced to β-subunit. Tyrosine kinase activity is activated and β-subunit is autophosphorylated, and insulin signaling commences
- The insulin receptor gene carries 12 exons and generates two isoforms—IRa and IRb—through alternate splicing of exon 11. The IRa retains exon 11 and has molecular affinity for both insulin and insulin-like growth factor-2 while IRb omits exon 11 and has high affinity for insulin only (Fig. 8.2)
- To understand insulin signaling pathway, it is important to understand the following (Fig. 8.3):
  - Activated insulin receptor binds insulin receptor substrate (IRS) and phosphorylates it
  - Insulin receptor substrate is activated and it can activate several pathways

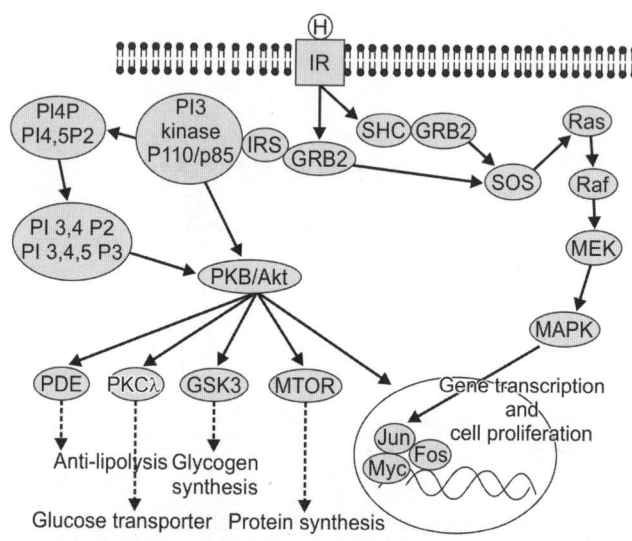

FIG. 8.3: Signal transduction for insulin

- Activated receptor initiates the inositol triphosphate/guanosine phosphate (IP_3/DAG) pathway by activating phospholipase Cγ (PLCγ). Src homology domains (SH2 domains) of PLCγ bind to specific tyrosines of the activated receptors and position the enzyme (PLCγ) close to membrane bound PIP2. Activated insulin receptor also phosphorylates tyrosine residues of PLCγ and thus enhances its hydrolase activity to produce IP_3/DAG
- Activated insulin receptor also initiates another phosphoinositide pathway, the phosphatidylinositol-3 kinase pathway (PI_3 kinase pathway). Several PI_3 kinases are known. The best characterized has two subunits, a P110 subunit with catalytic activity and P85 subunit with an SH2 domain

- Just like PLCγ, SH2 domain of PI3 binds to phosphotyrosines of activated insulin receptor and PI_3 K's catalytic subunit produces PI3, 4-biphosphate or PI3,4,5 triphosphate. These PI3 phosphates transduce several signaling pathways
- The primary binding target of PI_3 phosphates is protein kinase B (PKB or Akt), a serine/threonine kinase. PI3 also has two domains, a kinase domain and a pH domain. pH domain tightly binds the 3-phosphate in both PI3,4 biphosphate and PI3,4,5 triphosphate. This results into activation of PI3K by removal of inhibition of the catalytic site by the pH domain in the cytosol. However, PI3K is only partially activated. For full activation, it recruits another kinase phosphoinositide-dependent kinase-1 (PDK-1) to the plasma membrane via binding of its pH domain to the PI-3 phosphates. PDK-I phosphorylates PKB on one serine residue to activate PKB. Phosphorylation of another Serine residue is necessary to fully activate PKB
- Activated PKB I:
  - Stimulates GLUT4 translocation from cytoplasm to plasma membrane to increase glucose transport in muscle and adipose tissue
  - In liver and muscles stimulates glycogen synthase to increase glycogenesis. Fully activated PKB dissociates from plasma membrane and phosphorylates its several target proteins.

Insulin Receptor Substrate

Insulin receptor substrate is a protein which contains a phosphotyrosine binding domain. As their name indicates they can bind proteins like insulin and IGF. On binding the hormone, they get phosphorylated and become active. At least 4 IRS are known and IRS 1 and IRS 2 are important for response to insulin and IGF. Insulin receptor substrate proteins are a family of cytoplasmic adapter proteins that serve as bridge between the insulin receptor and the downstream signaling molecules. The IRS1 and IRS2 are ubiquitously expressed whereas IRS4 is primarily restricted to brain, kidneys, liver, and thymus. Although these proteins share significant homology, the phenotypes of knockout mice suggest that IRS proteins have non-redundant normal functions. These proteins carry no intrinsic enzyme activity.

GLUCOSE TRANSPORTERS

These are a wide group of membrane proteins that help in the transport of glucose through the plasma membrane. These are facilitative GLUTs and use diffusion gradient to transport glucose. At least 12 are known. The GLUT-4 is found in adipose tissue, liver, and striated muscles and helps in the insulin regulated glucose transport. The GLUT-5 is important in the transport of fructose. Three classes of GLUTs have been described.

Sodium-dependent glucose transporters (SGLT1 and SGLT2): These are members of a larger family of sodium transporters encoded by *SLCSA* gene. They utilize electrochemical gradient of Na^+ to pump glucose against concentration gradient. The SGLT1 is mostly distributed in the intestine and distal collecting tubule of the kidneys and SGLT2 is dominantly found in the proximal convoluted tubule of the kidneys.

GLUCAGON

It is a 29 amino acid peptide hormone secreted by α cells of islets of Langerhans of pancreas. It has a molecular weight of 3485 Daltons. It is synthesized as proglucagon in (α cells) of islets and converted to glucagon by enzyme pro-protein convertase. Its secretion is regulated by circulating concentrations of glucose.

Functions

Its function is opposite to insulin. It increases blood glucose levels by way of promoting glycogenolysis of liver glycogen. Glucagon is secreted in response to low blood glucose levels. Its secretion is inhibited by hyperglycemia, insulin, somatostatin, and GLP-1. Fatty acids and amino acids stimulate its secretion. Glucose enters α cells via GLUT1 transporter and suppresses glucagon secretion. Failure to suppress glucagon is a cardinal feature to type 2 diabetes mellitus.

Mechanism of Action

Its receptor is a G-protein coupled receptor. On binding glucagon, there is a conformational change in the receptor which activates G-proteins which in turn activate adenylate cyclase. Adenylate cyclase converts ATP to cAMP which activates protein kinase A (PKA). Activated PKA activates phosphorylase kinase which phosphorylates glycogen phosphorylase converting into its active form phosphorylase A which releases glucose-phosphate from glycogen. Epinephrine exactly functions in the same manner but on muscle glycogen. Major function of glucagon is to regulate glucose homeostasis through its action in the liver. While it stimulates gluconeogenesis, it inhibits activity of glycogen synthase at the same time. Glucagon is intimately involved in the genesis of ketoacidosis. Glucagon also has a role mediated by the receptors found in hypothalamus.

Glucagon also promotes lipolysis breaking triacylglycerol (triglycerides) into fatty acids which are used as fuel by cells in the body. This is achieved by activation of PKA which subsequently activates lipases in adipose tissue.

SOMATOSTATIN

It is a unique hormone which is synthesized and secreted by more than one gland/organ. It is synthesized in hypothalamus, pancreas, stomach, and intestine. In all vertebrates there are six somatostatin genes named SS1 to SS6. However, in humans there is only one somatostatin gene named SST. It is also unique as it exists in two forms, one composed of 14 amino acids and a second of 28 amino acids.

Somatostatin produced in hypothalamus is carried to the anterior pituitary where it inhibits the secretion of growth hormone. Thus, it is called growth hormone inhibiting hormone or somatotropin release-inhibiting factor. Its secretion is under negative feedback control. In all the glands/organs its role is inhibitory. It inhibits release of growth hormone as described above but via inhibiting the release of growth hormone–releasing hormone. It also inhibits the release of thyroid stimulating hormone and prolactin.

In pancreas, it is produced by D cells and inhibits the release of insulin and glucagon from adjacent β cells and α cells thus having a paracrine role. In gastrointestinal tract tract, it suppresses the release of the following gastrointestinal hormones:
- Gastrin
- Cholecystokinin
- Secretin
- Motilin
- Vasoactive intestinal polypeptide
- Gastric inhibitory peptide
- Enteroglucagon.

In kidney, it inhibits the secretion of renin.

Somatostatin 28: In gastrointestinal tract, it is the major somatostatin. It has the biological activity of somatostatin 14 but has a 14 amino acid extension at the N-terminus.

PANCREATIC POLYPEPTIDE

It is a 36 amino acid hormone secreted by F cells of islets of Langerhans of pancreas. Its molecular weight is 4,200 Da. Its C-terminal tyrosine is animated. It is synthesized as 95 amino acid prepropancreatic polypeptide. Its secretion is increased after a protein meal, fasting, exercise, and acute hypoglycemia. Somatostatin inhibits its secretion. Its plasma levels are elevated in anorexia nervosa. Its secretion is augmented in hormonal active pancreatic tumors and gastrinomas.

Function: It regulates both the exocrine and endocrine secretion of pancreas thus, acting in a paracrine manner.

AMYLIN

It is also called islet amyloid polypeptide (IAPP). It is co-secreted with insulin from the β cells of islets in a ratio of 100 to 1. It is processed from a 89 residue pre-pro IAPP which has a 22 residue N-terminal signal peptide. It forms a 67 residue pro-amylin which is converted to mature 37 amino acid residues IAPP.

Its overall effect is to slow the rate of glucose appearance in the blood after a meal. This is achieved via coordinate slowing down gastric emptying, inhibition of secretion of gastric juice, pancreatic and bile ejection, and a resulting reduction in food intake. It also inhibits glucagon secretion thus inhibiting gluconeogenesis. Amylin has been linked with type 2 diabetes and loss of islet β cells. Although the role of amylin in the development of type 2 diabetes is still unclear, the pancreas of 95% of type 2 diabetics contain amyloid deposits of amylin. These deposits increase in amount with the severity of the disease. Interestingly mouse amylin which differs from human amylin by 6 amino acids does not form amyloids.

ENDOCRINE PANCREATIC DISORDERS

Diabetes Mellitus

Diabetes mellitus (diabetes) is characterized by high circulating blood glucose (hyperglycemia) with glucose spillage into urine (glycosuria). Normal fasting blood glucose levels in human is 70–100 mg/dL and approximately 140 mg/dL in postprandial condition (2 h after meal). Body defends these levels very vigorously to provide energy to nervous tissue and erythrocytes [red blood cells (RBCs)] which get almost 100% energy from glucose only. Blood glucose level increases either due to absolute or relative deficiency of insulin. As mentioned earlier, the first and foremost function of insulin is to increase utilization of glucose, thus in deficient insulin conditions glucose level increases.

Absolute insulin deficiency occurs due to destruction of β cells of islet of Langerhans, the reason usually is autoimmune destruction of β cells. It occurs in early life and the patient requires insulin to maintain stable glucose levels. This condition is called type 1 diabetes (previously called insulin dependent diabetes). This condition is prevalent in only 5–10% of total patients of diabetes. In relative deficiency of insulin, the insulin secreted by the patient is not sufficient to maintain normal blood glucose level. The reason could be insulin resistance/pancreatic dysfunction. This condition is called type 2 diabetes (previously called noninsulin dependent diabetes). With time these patients might require insulin. Heredity plays a major role in this condition though the condition is multifactorial. Type 2 diabetes is mostly found in persons above the age of 35 years. These days it is also found increasingly in younger patients as well. Insulin resistance is an important component and with passage of time there is progressive worsening of β cell failure.

Prediabetes: This is a condition in which if a person's fasting blood glucose level is more than 100–125, the person is likely to have diabetes after about 10 years. It is a precursor to diabetes. Life style intervention (healthy diet/weight loss and exercise) are very effective in reducing/delaying progression to full blown type 2 diabetes mellitus.

Certain medications have added role in delaying the onset of diabetes and these include thiazolidinedione (insulin sensitizer) and metformin.

Rare forms of diabetes: A number of much rare monogenic conditions result in nonautoimmune diabetes. The most notable is maturity onset diabetes (MODY). It has autosomal dominant inheritance and presents with nonketotic hyperglycemia due to β cell failure. As the name indicates, it occurs in younger groups between the ages of 6 months and 35 years of age. Currently, 12 subtypes are recognized, and 13 genes implicated. Depending on the disease subtype, patients with MODY have different disease trajectories. Other rare form is the neonatal diabetes mellitus typically presenting before 6 months of age, and syndromic diabetes (Wolfram syndrome, Wolcott-Rallison syndrome), and mitochondrial diabetes associated with mutation in maternal mitochondrial DNA.

Gestational diabetes: It is a condition in which women without previously diagnosed diabetes have high blood glucose levels during pregnancy. It is a state of insulin resistance. Mothers suffering from gestational diabetes give birth to overweight babies. Unless there is a previous history, typically diagnosis is made between 24 and 28th week of gestation following a glucose tolerance test. In most case dietary management is sufficient, but if hyperglycemia is pronounced oral insulin secretagogue (sulfonylureas) or insulin may be required. Metformin has been used as well.

Diabetes complications: Chronic elevation of blood glucose level leads to damage of blood vessels. The endothelial cells lining the blood vessels are exposed to more glucose than normal. This leads to formation of more glycoproteins and cause the basement membrane to grow thicker and weaker which results both in microvascular and macrovascular complications. These complications are retinopathy (eye disease), nephropathy (renal disease), neuropathy (disease of nervous system), and diabetic cardiomyopathy. This is a very broad topic and scope of this book does not allow discussing it in detail. However, diabetes mellitus and its complications is one of the major causes of human mortality worldwide.

Glycated Hemoglobin

Glycation of proteins is a normal phenomenon. In case of hemoglobin, a nonenzymatic reaction attaches glucose to end terminal valine of β-chain of hemoglobin. As the blood glucose levels rise as in case of diabetes, glucose molecules attach to hemoglobin in RBCs and do not detach. A buildup of glycosylated hemoglobin (HbA1c) within the RBCs, therefore, reflects the average levels of glucose to which the RBC has been exposed during its life time of 120 days. Measuring HbA1c reflects the average level of glucose in the last 2–3 months. The increased levels of HbA1c thus, reflect poor control of diabetes. A value of 6% of HbA1c is considered good control and a value of 10 or above shows poor control. A 1% decrease in HbA1c decreases the risk of diabetic complications of type 1 diabetes or type 2 diabetes by 25%.

Reference range of HbA1c:
- Below 6.0%: Normal value
- 6.0–7.0%: Good control
- 7.0–8.0%: Fair control
- 8.0–10.0%: Unsatisfactory control
- Above 10%: Poor control.

Hypoglycemia

It implies low blood sugar. A value of less than 70 mg/dL of blood glucose is considered low blood glucose. It is very dangerous condition and a person can have convulsions due to low blood glucose because brain does not get energy. Its major reason is excessive insulin either due to an insulinoma of β cells or excessive dose of insulin, or oral drugs used to control diabetes. It is treated by administering orally glucose (10-20 g), whereas in severe cases an injection of glucagon is given which will cause glycogenolysis and gluconeogenesis, and thus raise blood glucose levels. People with unprovoked and spontaneous hypoglycemia should be investigated for insulin secreting pancreatic tumor (insulinoma). Patients generally meet criteria for Whipple Triad—documentation of hypoglycemia (BG <50 mgs/dL); symptoms of hypoglycemia disappear after administration of glucose.

APPLIED ASPECTS

Understanding of glucose metabolism and role of insulin and glucagon in its regulation is very important for endocrinologists taking care of patients with diabetes mellitus or pancreatogenic hypoglycemia. There are several diagnostic criteria and diagnostic tools (tests) that help in identifying the disease and making correct diagnosis. It is beyond the scope of this book to address diagnosis and testing methodologies in detail. Adequate details have been provided about insulin release and mechanism of insulin action.

Insulin resistance and insulin sensitivity have occupied central stage not only in pathogenesis of diabetes mellitus, but also topics related to aging and cancer. In coming years, we shall learn more about these connections and hopefully as better understanding emerges, we could be closer to finding cures.

New connections are emerging from studies of gut microbiome and the insulin resistance, and it opens up new opportunities for treatment of diabetes mellitus.

9
CHAPTER

Gonads

Gonads (testes in males and ovaries in females) are primary sex organs having dual function of synthesizing sex hormones and producing germ cells. Sex hormones are steroid in nature and cause growth, development, and maintenance of reproductive system. Sex hormones are of three main types:
1. Androgens: These are male sex hormones and are C-19 steroids
2. Estrogens: They are female sex hormones and C-18 steroids in which ring A is phenolic in nature. These are predominantly ovarian hormones produced by ovarian follicles and corpus luteum of the ovary
3. Progesterone: It is C-21 female sex hormone produced in the luteal phase of menstrual cycle by corpus luteum. It is also produced in smaller amounts by adrenal cortex.

ANDROGEN BIOSYNTHESIS

Androgens produced in the testes are actually synthesized by the interstitial cells (Leydig cells). Cholesterol, the precursor for androgen synthesis is transported into mitochondria where it is acted upon by side chain cleavage enzyme P450scc to form pregnenolone. This reaction is promoted by luteinizing hormone (LH). The biosynthesis of testosterone from pregnenolone either involves Δ^5 (dehydroepiandrosterone) pathway or Δ^4 (progesterone) pathway.

- The Δ^4 (progesterone) pathway is shown on the right side of figure 9.1. Pregnenolone is initially converted into progesterone by enzymes 3β-OHSD and $\Delta^{5,4}$-isomerase. Enzymes 17α-hydroxylase and 17, 20-lyase (residing in a single protein) convert progesterone into 17-hydroxyprogesterone and then into androstenedione. The latter is converted into testosterone in the presence of enzyme 17β-OHSD
- The Δ5 (dehydroepiandrosterone) pathway is shown on the left side of figure 9.1. Enzymes 17α-hydroxylase and 17, 20-lyase (residing in a single protein) convert pregnenolone into 17-hydroxypregnenolone and then into dehydroepiandrosterone. The latter is converted into androstenediol by enzyme 17β-OHSD. Testosterone is formed from androstenediol in the presence of enzymes 3β-OHSD and $\Delta^{5,4}$-isomerase.

Testosterone produced in the testes is acted upon by enzyme 5α-reductase in target tissues to form potent metabolite, dihydrotestosterone (DHT). Thus, testosterone may be regarded as a prohormone. About 400 μg of DHT is produced daily and its level is about one-tenth of that of testosterone.

Androgens-biochemical Functions

- They help in the development of male secondary sexual characteristics. They also help in the growth and development of male reproductive organs
- They help in the process of spermatogenesis
- They cause positive nitrogen balance by promoting protein synthesis and thus increasing muscle mass
- They promote growth of bones before closure of epiphyseal cartilage.

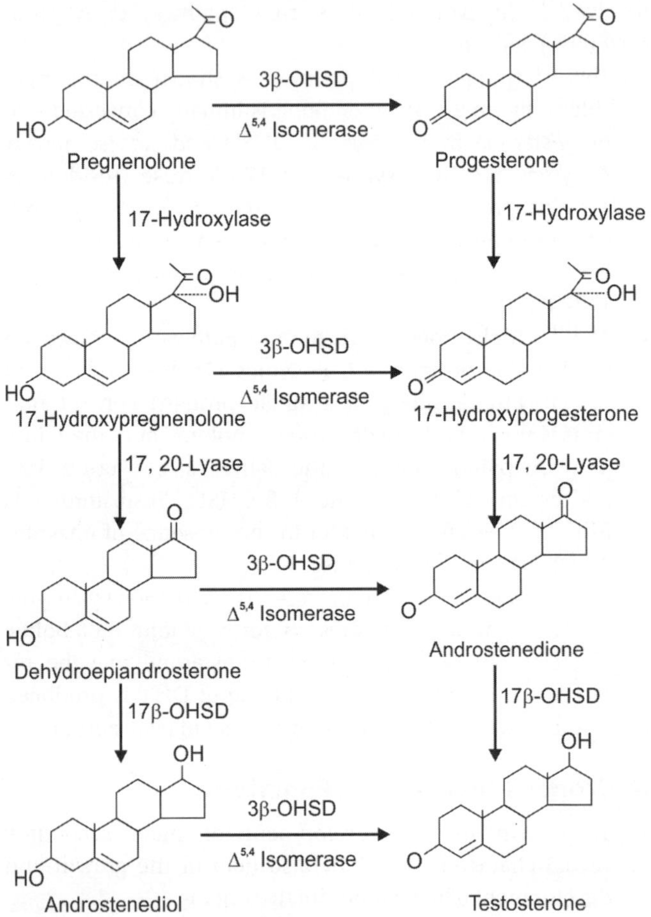

FIG. 9.1: Testosterone synthesis

Mechanism of Action of Testosterone

Testosterone acts by binding to its androgen receptor in the cytoplasm of target tissue cells or it can be reduced to 5α-DHT. Dihydrotestosterone binds to the androgen receptor more strongly than testosterone and thus is about 10 times more potent than testosterone. The ligand receptor complex undergoes a structural change and enters nucleus where it binds to hormone response element (HREs) of deoxyribonucleic acid (DNA) causing transcription of certain genes, producing androgen effects. The bones and brain are two tissues on which testosterone acts after its conversion to estradiol. In bones estradiol accelerates ossification of cartilage to bone leading to closure of epiphysis. In brain, estradiol serve the most important feedback signal to the hypothalamus affecting LH secretion.

ESTROGEN BIOSYNTHESIS

Aromatization of androgens leads to the formation of estrogens. Estrogens include Estrone (E1), Estradiol (E2), and Estriol (E3).

Estrogen synthesis is under control of LH and follicle-stimulating hormone (FSH). All the estrogens can be synthesized by the placenta whereas ovary synthesizes only E_1 and E_2. Primary estrogen in humans is estradiol, synthesized in the ovary whereas during pregnancy more amount of estriol is produced. Aromatization of androgens in the presence of aromatase enzyme complex, results in the formation of estrogens. In the presence of this enzyme complex, testosterone and androstenedione (derived from theca cells of ovarian follicle) are converted into estradiol and estrone, (in granulosa cells of ovarian follicle), respectively (Fig. 9.2). Aromatase enzyme complex consists of P450 monooxygenase and catalyzes three hydroxylation steps, each step requiring O_2 and nicotinamide adenine dinucleotide phosphate. The activity of this enzyme is present in variety of tissues such as liver and skin.

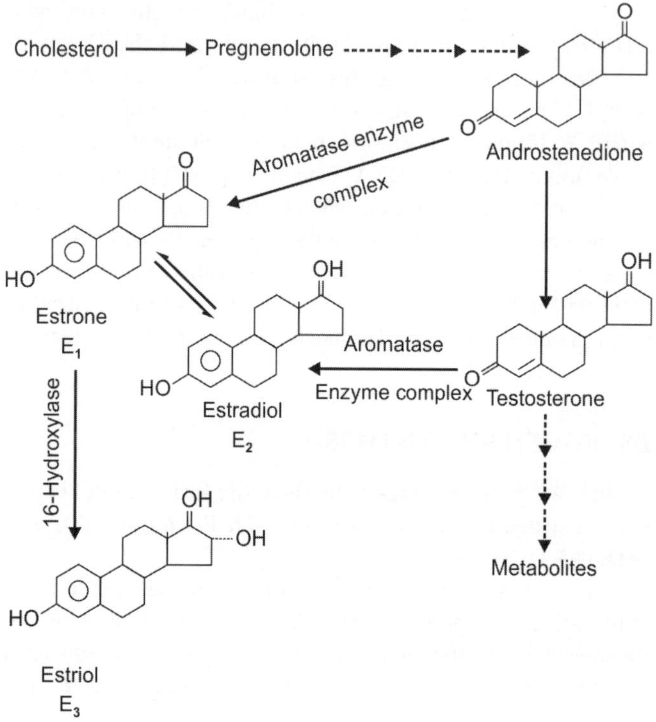

FIG. 9.2: Estrogen biosynthesis

Estrogens-biochemical Functions

- They promote growth and development of female reproductive organs and maintenance of menstrual cycle
- They promote the development of female secondary sexual characteristics
- They promote synthesis of lipids in the adipose tissue and this accounts for the fact that women have more fat than men

- They decrease incidence of atherosclerosis and coronary heart disease due to their hypocholesterolemic effect. They increase high-density lipoprotein fraction and decrease low-density lipoprotein fraction
- They promote protein synthesis in liver
- They promote bone calcification and growth, and in this way their function is similar to androgens.

Mechanism of Action of Estrogens

Estradiol receptors Erα and Erβ are located in the nucleus. Estradiol receptor complex binds HREs of DNA and regulates activity of different genes. Recently, estrogen receptors have been discovered on cell membranes which mediate a variety of non-genomic effects.

PROGESTERONE BIOSYNTHESIS

Progesterone is produced by corpus luteum in the ovary and placenta. Progesterone is secreted by corpus luteum as an end product as it lacks enzymes necessary to convert progesterone to other steroid hormones. Progesterone is also synthesized in the adrenal gland and testes in males where it is precursor for the synthesis of other steroid hormones.

Progesterone-biochemical Functions

- It is essential for the process of implantation and maintenance of pregnancy (pregnancy hormone)
- It stimulates the development of uterus and mammary gland
- By an unknown mechanism, it is also known to increase the body temperature.

Activin

Activin is a dimer of two similar or identical β-subunits linked by a single disulphide bond. It is of three types:
1. Activin AB which is formed of $β_A$ and $β_B$ subunits
2. Activin B is formed of two $β_B$ subunits
3. Activin A is formed of two $β_A$ subunits.

It is produced in the gonads, pituitary, and the placenta. Its function is exactly opposite to inhibin. It increases FSH secretion. In the ovarian follicles, it increases FSH binding and FSH-induced aromatization. It increases testosterone synthesis and enhances LH action in the ovary and the testes. It also enhances spermatogenesis. Its mechanism of action is similar to inhibin.

Inhibin

As its name indicates, it is an inhibitory hormone. It inhibits the secretion of FSH both in males and females by negative feedback action. It is secreted by sertoli cells of testis in males and granulosa cells of ovaries in females. As described previously, it is a glycoprotein hormone formed of α- and β-subunits linked by a disulphide bond. It is of two types A and B. Inhibin A comprises an α-subunit and $β_A$ subunits whereas B has a $β_B$ subunit in place of $β_A$ subunit. These inhibins function at different times during menstrual cycle. Inhibin B reaches peak level in the early to mid follicular phase and reaches a second peak at ovulation. Inhibin A has maximum level in mid luteal phase.

Inhibin Receptors

They are cell surface receptors. These are dimers of serine-threonine kinase subunits that regulate cytoplasmic SMADs. The SMADs are intracellular proteins that transduce extra-cellular signals from transforming growth factor-β (TGF-β) and other similar ligands to the nucleus where they activate gene transcription. Thus, they act as transcription factors. Their name is derived as they are homologues to the drosophila proteins, mothers against decapentaplegic (MAD), and caenorhabditis elegans protein SMA (from gene sma for small body size). There are three classes of SMADs:

1. Receptor-regulated SMADs (R-SMAD): These include SMAD 1-3, 5, and 8/9
2. Common-mediated SMADs (Co-SMAD): SMAD-4—It interacts with R-SMADS to participate in signaling
3. Antagonistic SMADS: These include SMAD6-7. These inhibit activation of R and Co-SMAD.

Anti-Müllerian Hormone

Anti-Müllerian hormone (AMH) is a protein hormone in humans encoded by AMH gene. It inhibits the development of the Müllerian ducts in the male embryo. It is also called Müllerian inhibiting factor, Müllerian inhibitory substance (MIS), and Müllerian-inhibiting hormone. It is secreted by sertoli cells during embryogenesis. In the female, it is secreted by granulosa cells of ovarian follicles. It is a dimeric glycoprotein with a molecular weight of 140 kDa.

Anti-Müllerian hormone is produced by male fetus sertoli cells of the testis from the 5th to 8th week of embryogenesis and in females fetus is formed from 36th week of gestation in the granulosa cells of the ovaries. In 1940's AMH was known as "MIS" for its action on the Müllerian ducts. These ducts are named after Johannes Peter Müller, as he studied and traced the development of these ducts.

Anti-Müllerian hormone is a dimeric glycoprotein hormone and has structure similar to activin and inhibin, and belongs to the class of TGF-β family of proteins. It has a molecular weight of 140 KD.

Anti-Müllerian hormone assay in females: After puberty it controls the maturation of primary follicles (formation of ovum) by regulating the action of FSH on ovaries. The level of AMH is in direct proportion to the reserve of ovum. Its measurement is also important in females who wish to have *in vitro* fertilization (IVF). Women with normal or slightly elevated levels of AMH have shown to have successful IVF.

MENSTRUAL CYCLE

This cycle occurs in human females and varies between 25 and 35 days in length with an average of 28 days. This cycle can be divided into two main phases:

Follicular Phase

Under the influence of FSH, ovarian follicles begin to mature and start releasing estradiol. The latter reaches its peak value 24 hours before the peak values of LH and FSH. Luteinizing hormone peak results in ovulation (release of secondary oocyte from the ovary). In this phase, the levels of progesterone are low. This phase of menstrual cycle is not fixed and the variation of this phase causes observed variations in the length of menstrual cycle.

Luteal Phase

This phase of menstrual cycle is fixed (14 + 2 days). After ovulation, the ruptured follicular cells of ovarian follicle form corpus luteum which starts producing progesterone and estradiol. Progesterone is the predominant hormone of this phase which prepares the endometrium of uterus for implantation of the fertilized ovum. Luteinizing hormone released by anterior pituitary maintains corpus luteum for few days. If implantation does not take place, corpus luteum regresses and production of progesterone stops. In the absence

TABLE 1: Hormone levels during menstrual cycle

	FSH (mIU/mL)	LH (mIU/mL)	Estradiol (pg/mL)	17-OH Progesterone (ng/mL)
Follicular phase	2.5–10.2	1.9–12.5	19.5–144.2	0.20–1.30
Midcycle peak	3.4–33.4	8.7–76.3	63.9–356.7	–
Luteal phase	1.5–9.1	0.5–16.9	55.8–212.2	1.00–4.50
Prolactin levels			ng/mL	
Normally menstruating			2.8–29.2	
Pregnant			9.7–208.5	
Postmenopausal			1.8–20.3	

of progesterone, endometrium sheds resulting in menstruation. After this the new menstrual cycle begins.

If implantation occurs, human chorionic gonadotropin (hCG) released by the cells of implanted embryo maintain corpus luteum due to which synthesis of progesterone continues. Corpus luteum produces progesterone till placenta starts to make sufficient quantities of progesterone (Table 1).

PATHOPHYSIOLOGY OF REPRODUCTIVE SYSTEM

Primary hypogonadism: In males, it is due to testes dysfunction (decreased sperm production or decreased androgen secretion or both), whereas in females it is due to ovarian deficiency (decreased ovulation or decreased hormone production or both). If dysfunction occurs before puberty, secondary sexual characteristics do not develop. In such males, failure of testosterone secretion results in eunuchoidism. Due to deficiency of testosterone and abundance of estrogen, male mammary glands may show excessive development which results in gynecomastia. If testicular dysfunction develops postpubertally, there may be regression of some characteristic—testicular atrophy, baldness, reduced frequency of shaving, and reduction in muscle mass. Klinefelter syndrome and Turner's syndrome would be examples of this kind of hypogonadism.

Secondary hypogonadism: In both males and females, it is due to defective secretion of gonadotropins or impairment of gonadotropin releasing hormone (GnRH) secretion. Hypogonadism due to defects in GnRH secretion or damage to pituitary gland would be examples of secondary hypogonadism.

Turner's syndrome: It is chromosomal disorder in which the female has abnormal karyotype (44+XO). Such a female often presents with short stature, failure to menstruate, and typical phenotype. They have rudimentary ovaries, small uterus, and undeveloped mammary glands. These days such patients are treated with growth hormone and estrogen replacement to enhance height and induce secondary sex characteristics. There is higher risk for cardiac and renal malformations. They are also at risk for thyroid dysfunction and diabetes mellitus.

Klinefelter's syndrome: Male has abnormal phenotype (44+XXY). Such a male will have undeveloped firm testes, sparse body hair, and gynecomastia. It is widely underdiagnosed before puberty. Clinical presentation varies according to age. At the time of puberty these patients are generally of average or taller height. There may be deficits in certain domains of cognition mainly language and executive functions. Chromosome analysis in lymphocytes helps confirm the diagnosis. Leydig cell dysfunction is variable. These patients are at risk for diabetes mellitus, leg ulceration, and venous thromboembolism.

Kallmann syndrome: A relative rare reproductive disorder that is primarily caused by GnRH deficiency. Typically, it is associated with low circulating hormone levels of LH and FSH in conjunction with low levels of circulating sex steroids. About 50% cases suffer from aberrations of smell (absent sense of smell–anosmia or reduced sense of smell–hyposmia). It is then called Kallmann syndrome. There is developmental defect in migration of GnRH neurons as they travel in close association with olfactory neurons during embryogenesis.

Supermales and superfemales: Supermales have genotype 44+XYY and superfemales can have variable genotype (44+XXX or 44+XXXX etc.). In supermales, there is overproduction of male sex hormones due to which they become more aggressive. In superfemales, there is abnormal sexual development and mental retardation.

APPLIED ASPECTS

Sex steroids produced by the gonads are very important for phenotypic expression, pubertal development, and reproductive function(s). If there is deficiency of sex steroids prior to onset of puberty, puberty shall be delayed and epiphyseal closure of long bones delayed. Puberty shall have to be induced by provision of appropriate sex steroid. If the gonad is developmentally defective, injured, or damaged then the only recourse would be to provide the sex steroid of interest. If the gonad is intact then gonadotropins (LH, FSH), hCG, and GnRH would be on the menu of choices. In order for GnRH to work, pituitary must be intact.

Sex steroids work through their receptors. In normal males a single androgen receptor binds to both testosterone and DHT, but with higher affinity for DHT. In the absence of ligand, androgen receptor is located in the cytoplasm complexed to heat shock proteins and other chaperones. Binding of testosterone or DHT leads to shedding of chaperones and the complex rapidly translocates to the nucleus where it binds to genomic androgen response element. If the receptors are dysfunctional, a state of hypogonadism results, but sex steroid levels will remain elevated. Such a situation may be seen with defective androgen receptor mutations leading to androgen resistant state with female phenotype (testicular-feminization syndrome). A case of defective/mutated estrogen receptor (loss-of-function mutation in ER-α gene) (Estrogen resistance) was reported in a male patient in 1994. He had normal levels of plasma testosterone, but high levels of estrogen (for a male), LH, and FSH. He had incomplete epiphyseal fusion, and low bone mineral density. He also had features of insulin resistance and premature atherosclerosis.

Defects in conversion of testosterone to dihydrotestosterone (5α reductase type 2 deficiency) result in birth of male babies with ambiguous genitalia. These males virilize by age of 11–12 years.

Defective/excessive aromatase expressions have been recorded, and distinct syndromes with biochemical characterization reported. Patients with aromatase deficiency are unable to convert androgens to estrogens resulting in high circulating androgen levels with low circulating estrogen levels. Levels of LH and FSH are elevated owing to lack of estrogen negative feedback on hypothalamus. Aromatase deficiency is associated with a maternal history of virilization during pregnancy. Female babies are born with ambiguous genitalia.

10
CHAPTER

Adipose Tissue Hormones

Adipose tissue, especially white adipose tissue is a source of several hormones collectively called adipokines. The major hormones are leptin and adiponectin.

LEPTIN

Leptin is a 16 kDa polypeptide having 167 amino acids with structural homology to cytokines. Its precursor is 18 kDa protein which is cleaved to mature leptin of 16 kDa molecular weight. It was discovered in 1994. Adipocytes secrete leptin in direct proportion to mass of adipose tissue as well as induvidual's nutritional status. Several factors regulate leptin expression and secretion. For example, leptin secretion is increased by insulin, glucocorticoids, tumor necrosis factor-α (TNF-α), estrogens, and CCAAT/enhancer-binding protein-α and it is decreased by β3-adrenergic activity, androgens, growth hormone, and peroxisome proliferator-activated receptor-γ agonists.

The effects of leptin on energy homeostasis are well known. Many of its effects, particularly on energy intake and expenditure, are mediated via hypothalamic pathways, whereas other effects are mediated by direct action on peripheral tissues including muscle and pancreatic β cells. Although leptin is considered an anti-obesity hormone, its primary role is to serve as a metabolic signal of energy sufficiency rather than excess. Leptin levels decline rapidly with caloric restriction and weight loss. This decline is associated with adaptive physiological responses to starvation including increased appetite and decreased energy expenditure. These effects have been observed in leptin-deficient mice and humans, despite massive obesity.

Leptin Receptors

Leptin receptors are expressed in both the central nervous system and periphery and these are members of the cytokine receptor class I superfamily. Although several splice variants of the leptin receptor have been identified, the long form mediates the majority of leptin's myriad effects.

Functions of Leptin

The mechanism for leptin resistance is unknown but may result from defects in leptin signaling or transport across the blood-brain barrier. Clearly, the most sensitive portion of the leptin dose-response curve resides in the physiological range between the low levels induced by food restriction and the rising levels induced by refeeding, and not in the supraphysiological range associated with obesity. This role of leptin as an indicator of energy sufficiency makes sense from an evolutionary perspective but provides no consolation in our current environment of energy abundance. Other main functions of leptin include:
- Leptin regulates neuroendocrine function and traditional endocrine systems. Leptin deficiency in Lep^{ob}/Lep^{ob} mice activates hypothalamic-pituitary-adrenal (HPA) axis and suppresses the hypothalamic-pituitary-thyroid and gonadal axis

- Leptin decreases hypercortisolemia in Lep^{ob}/Lep^{ob} mice, inhibits stress-induced secretion of hypothalamic corticotropin-releasing hormone in mice, and inhibits cortisol secretion from rodent and human adrenocortical cells *in vitro*. The role of leptin in HPA activity in humans *in vivo* remains unclear
- Leptin hastens puberty in normal mice and restores normal gonadotropin secretion, and reproductive function in humans and leptin-deficient mice
- Suppressed thyroid hormone levels are normalized by leptin in leptin-deficient mice and humans, in part via stimulation of thyrotropin-releasing hormone (TRH) expression and secretion from hypothalamic TRH neurons
- Leptin also has direct effects via peripheral leptin receptors in the ovary, testis, prostate, and placenta
- Leptin regulates immune function, hematopoiesis, angiogenesis, and bone development
- Leptin replacement during fasting prevents starvation-induced changes in the hypothalamic-pituitary-gonadal and thyroid axes in healthy men
- Leptin helps in proliferation and differentiation of hematopoietic cells, stimulates endothelial cell growth, alters cytokine production by immune cells, and angiogenesis, and accelerates wound healing
- Leptin normalizes the suppressed immune function associated with leptin deficiency and malnutrition
- Leptin helps in bone development as leptin-deficient Lep^{ob}/Lep^{ob} mice increase bone mass, despite hypercortisolemia and hypogonadism. It is believed that the ventral medial hypothalamus (VMH) is involved in leptin's effect on bone mass. Leptin-responsive neurons in the VMH are known to influence sympathetic nervous system (SNS) activity. Leptin can decrease bone mass indirectly via activation of the SNS.

Clearly, leptin has diverse endocrine function in addition to its effects on energy homeostasis. Leptin is thus a major adipose tissue-derived endocrine hormone.

ADIPONECTIN

Adiponectin is known as adipose most abundant gene transcript 1 gelatin binding protein of 28 kDa, and adipocyte complement-related protein of 30 kDa. It is specifically expressed in differentiated adipocytes and circulates at high levels in the bloodstream. Adiponectin is an approximately 30 kDa, 244 amino acid polypeptide (encoded by ADIPOQ gene) containing an N-terminal signal sequence, a variable domain, a collagen-like domain, and a C-terminal globular domain. It shares strong sequence homology with type VIII and X collagen and complement component C1q. On determining the tertiary structure of the globular protein, it is observed that it bears a striking similarity to TNF-α, despite a lack of homology in primary sequence. Posttranslational modification by hydroxylation and glycosylation produces multiple isoforms, which assemble into trimers. The latter can then form higher-order oligomeric structures. A proteolytic cleavage product containing the globular domain of adiponectin also circulates at physiologically significant levels which has biological activity.

Adiponectin secreted into the bloodstream accounts for approximately 0.01% of all plasma protein. Its plasma concentration is around 5–10 µg/mL. Levels of adiponectin are reduced in diabetics compared to nondiabetics. Weight loss significantly increases circulating levels. Plasma concentrations reveal a sexual dimorphism, with females having higher levels as compared to males.

A strong and consistent inverse association between adiponectin and both insulin resistance and inflammatory states has been established. Plasma adiponectin declines before the occurrence of obesity and insulin resistance in primates which is indicative of the fact that lesser concentration of this hormone (hypoadiponectinemia) contributes to the pathogenesis of these conditions. Adiponectin levels are low with insulin resistance either due to obesity or lipodystrophy, and administration of adiponectin improves these metabolic conditions. Or one can say that adiponectin levels increase when insulin sensitivity improves, as it occurs after weight reduction or treatment with insulin-sensitizing drugs. Furthermore, several polymorphisms in the adiponectin gene are associated with obesity and insulin resistance. These epidemiological findings are supported by studies in murine models with altered adiponectin expression.

Adiponectin Receptors

Adiponectin receptor 1 and adiponectin receptor 2 are two main receptors and these contain seven-transmembrane domains which are structurally and functionally distinct from G-protein coupled receptors. Adiponectin receptor 1 is expressed mainly in muscle and functions as a high-affinity receptor for globular adiponectin and a low-affinity receptor for full-length adiponectin. Adiponectin receptor 2 is expressed mainly in liver and functions as an intermediate-affinity receptor for both globular and full-length adiponectin. The biological effects of adiponectin depend on relative circulating concentrations and properties of the different adiponectin isoforms and on the tissue-specific expression of the adiponectin receptor subtypes.

Adiponectin Functions

- Within the vascular wall, it inhibits monocyte adhesion by decreasing expression of adhesion molecules, inhibits

macrophage transformation to foam cells by inhibiting expression of scavenger receptors, and decreases proliferation of migrating smooth muscle cells in response to growth factors
- In liver, adiponectin enhances insulin sensitivity, decreases influx of nonesterified fatty acids, reduces hepatic glucose output, and increases fatty acid oxidation. In muscle, adiponectin stimulates glucose use and fatty acid oxidation
- Adiponectin increases nitric oxide production in endothelial cells and stimulate angiogenesis. These effects are mediated by increased phosphorylation of the insulin receptor, activation of cyclic adenosine monophosphate-activated protein kinase, and modulation of the nuclear factor kappa B pathway
- These functions indicate that adiponectin is a unique adipocyte-derived hormone with antidiabetic, antiatherogenic, and anti-inflammatory effects.

CHAPTER 11

Pineal Gland

Pineal gland is located in the brain. Its shape is of a pine cone, hence, the name pineal. In adult humans, it is about 0.8 cm long and weighs approximately 0.1 g. Pineal gland is relatively larger in children and begins to shrink with the onset of puberty. The gland is a source of the hormone melatonin, a derivative of tryptophan. The cells which produce this hormone are called pinealocytes.

In humans and other animals, in addition to secretion of melatonin, the gland produces several neuropeptides and neurotransmitters such as somatostatin, norepinephrine, and serotonin.

The secretion of melatonin is increased by sympathetic nervous system stimulation. Its secretion increases in dark and decreases in light. Thus, its major function is to regulate circadian rhythms (sleep cycles). In animals, it has been shown to block the secretion of gonadotropin releasing hormone by the hypothalamus, thus resulting into decreased secretion of luteinizing hormone and follicle stimulating hormone by the pituitary.

MECHANISM OF ACTION

In humans, there are two subtypes of melatonin receptors (MT1 and MT2) which bind melatonin. These are G-protein coupled receptors. The MT1 receptors are expressed in many regions of central nervous system (CNS) including hypothalamus. These are also expressed in many other organs and tissues such as retina, ovary, testis, mammary gland, aorta, gall bladder, liver, kidney, skin, and the immune system. The MT2 receptors are mostly expressed in CNS and some other tissues.

Melatonin binding to MT1 receptors inhibits adenylyl cyclase, thus producing less cyclic adenosine monophosphate (cAMP) which inhibits protein kinase A. This results into inhibition of phosphorylation of cAMP responsive element binding protein (CREB binding protein) into p-CREB. Binding of melatonin to MT1 receptors also activates phospholipase C (PLC). The latter affects ion channels and regulates ion flux inside the cell. Binding of melatonin to MT2 receptors inhibits both adenylyl cyclase and guanylyl cyclase, and also affects PLC.

12 CHAPTER

Gastrointestinal Tract Hormones

Gastrointestinal tract (GIT) is the richest source of hormones. It secretes about 50 hormones. In fact, first hormone secretin was discovered from GIT only by Bayliss and Starling in 1902. The list of GIT hormones which play some significant role is given in the introductory chapter.

SECRETIN

It is synthesized as a prohormone of 120 amino acids which has a signal peptide, spacer and secretin, and C-terminal peptide. It is a polypeptide of 27 amino acids and is secreted by the duodenum. Its major function is to stimulate the acinar cells of the pancreas to secrete water and bicarbonate into the pancreatic ducts that drain into the duodenum where water and bicarbonate neutralize the hydrochloric acid (HCl) secreted by the stomach. Secretin also inhibits the secretion of gastrin which stimulates the initial release of HCl into the stomach. Sequence of secretin is His-Ser-Asp-Gly-Thr-Phe-Thr-Ser-Glu-Leu-Ser-Arg-Leu-Arg-Asp-Ser-Ala-Arg-Leu-Gln-Arg-Leu-Leu-Gln-Gly-Leu-Val-NH$_2$.

Mechanism of Action

Its receptor is a G-protein coupled receptor. On binding of secretin to its receptor, adenylyl cyclase is activated increasing the formation of cyclic adenosine monophosphate which acts as a second messenger.

CHOLECYSTOKININ

It is a polypeptide hormone. It is also synthesized as prepro-cholecystokinin. It is composed of a varying number of amino acids depending on post-translational modification of *CCK* gene product. Three forms of *CCK* are known. These are *CCK58*, *CCK33*, and *CCK8*. It is secreted by the I-cells in the mucosal epithelium of small intestine. The presence of fatty acids and/or amino acids in the chyme entering the duodenum stimulates its release. Sequence of CCK8 is D-Y-M-G-W-M-D-F.

Its major function is to mediate digestion in the small intestine by inhibiting gastric emptying and HCl secretion. It stimulates pancreas to release digestive enzymes. It stimulates the contraction of gall bladder resulting into the delivery of bile into duodenum, thus, helping in emulsification of fats aiding their digestion and absorption.

GASTRIN

It is a polypeptide hormone of 17 amino acids. It also exists as gastrin 34 (big gastrin) and gastrin 14 (mini gastrin). It is produced by G-cells of the duodenum and in the pyloric antrum of the stomach. It is also produced by pancreas. Sequence of gastrin is X-G-P-W-L-E-E-E-E-E-A-Y-G-W-M-D-F.

Biochemical Functions

Gastrin stimulates parietal cells to stimulate HCl secretion directly or indirectly by binding onto CCK2/gastrin receptors on enterochromaffin-like cells of stomach. Enterochromaffin-like cells respond by releasing histamine which acts in a paracrine manner on parietal cells to stimulate secretion of H^+ ions. It also causes secretion of pepsinogen. Gastrin also induces pancreatic secretions and gall bladder emptying.

In Zollinger-Ellison syndrome, gastrin is produced in excessive amounts by a gastrinoma (mostly benign) of the duodenum or the pancreas.

VASOACTIVE INTESTINAL PEPTIDE

It is a peptide hormone of 28 amino acids. It is produced in gut, pancreas, and hypothalamus. It is synthesized as a prohormone having a 22 amino acid signal peptide. In GIT, it seems to induce smooth muscle relaxation, secretion of water into pancreatic juice and bile, and inhibits the secretion and absorption from the intestinal lumen. It also stimulates the pepsinogen secretion. It is a potent stimulator of prolactin as well.

GLUCAGON-LIKE PEPTIDE-1

It is a polypeptide derived from its precursor proglucagon. It is produced by the L-cells of the intestine. Its biologically active forms are glucagon-like peptide (GLP)-1-(7-37) and GLP-I-(7-36) NH_2. Its release is stimulated by nutrients such as carbohydrates, proteins, and lipids in the lumen of small intestine. It has a half-life of less than 2 minutes in the circulation. Its function is to decrease blood glucose level by increasing glucose-dependent insulin release (acts as an incretin hormone) and by inhibiting glucagon secretion. It also inhibits β cell apoptosis and stimulates the proliferation and differentiation of β cells of the islet of Langerhans. It also inhibits gastric secretion and motility. Its decreased secretion may contribute to the development of obesity and increased secretion may be responsible for postprandial reactive hypoglycemia.

GLUCAGON-LIKE PEPTIDE-2

It is a 33 amino acid polypeptide, also produced by the L-cells of the small intestine. It is cosecreted with GLP-1 on nutrient stimulation. It maintains the integrity of intestinal mucosal epithelium via effects on gastric motility and nutrient absorption.

GASTRIC INHIBITORY PEPTIDE

It is also called glucose-dependent insulinotropic peptide. It has 42 amino acids. It is synthesized as a 153 amino acid prohormone by K-cells of the mucosa of duodenum and jejunum. It is a true hormone in the sense that it is transported by blood. It functions to induce insulin secretion which is stimulated primarily by hyperosmolality of glucose in the duodenum. In adipocytes, it stimulates lipoprotein lipase activity which affects fatty acid metabolism. It acts through G-protein-coupled receptors found on β-cells of pancreas. It also inhibits HCl secretion in the stomach. This hormone falls under the category of incretin.

MOTILIN

It is a 22 amino acid peptide hormone (molecular weight 2,698 Dalton) which is secreted by M-cells of duodenum and jejunum. It activates gastric activity and thus, was named motilin. It also stimulates pepsin production and release of pancreatic polypeptide, and somatostatin from pancreas.

BOMBESIN

It is a 14 amino acid peptide hormone produced in gut and brain. It is also called neuromedin B and gastrin releasing peptide. It stimulates gastrin release from G-cells. It also stimulates the release of pancreatic enzymes and causes contraction of gall bladder. Bombesin receptors are G-protein-coupled receptors and these are of three types BBR1, BBR2, and BBR3.

GHRELIN

In the list of hormones, ghrelin seems to be the latest addition. It was discovered in 1999 after its receptor was discovered in 1996. Surprisingly, its counter, leptin, was also discovered in 1994. It is 28 amino acid peptide hormone and is synthesized as a 117 amino acid preproghrelin. Preproghrelin is converted into proghrelin and then to mature hormone. The cells that produce ghrelin are found mainly in the stomach and duodenum. These cells are also found in jejunum, lungs, islets, gonads, adrenal cortex, placenta, and kidney. Ghrelin is also called "hunger hormone". Ghrelin receptor is a G-protein-coupled receptor.

Functions of Ghrelin

Ghrelin participates in a complex process of "energy homeostasis", which adjusts both energy input by adjusting hunger signals and energy output by adjusting the proportion of energy going to adenosine triphosphate production, fat storage and short-term heat signals, and energy output, e.g., when the stomach is empty, ghrelin is secreted and when full, secretion stops. It acts via hypothalamus to increase hunger and to increase HCl secretion and gastrointestinal mobility to prepare the body for food intake. In this way, ghrelin is involved in the maintenance of body weight. When a person loses weight, ghrelin levels increase and vice versa. It functions exactly opposite to the adipose tissue hormone leptin.

PEPTIDE YY

It is a 36 amino acid peptide hormone of GIT first isolated from small intestine. As we know, Y is a symbol of amino acid tyrosine. Thus, the name peptide YY has been derived because it has tyrosines both at its N and C terminals. Its major functions are:
- Vasoconstriction
- Inhibition of gastric acid secretion
- Reduction of pancreatic and intestinal secretions
- Inhibition of gastrointestinal motility.

13
CHAPTER

Hormones from Liver

Liver produces:
- Insulin-like growth factor-1 (IGF-1)
- Insulin-like growth factor-2 (IGF-2)

INSULIN-LIKE GROWTH FACTOR 1

It is called IGF because its structure is like insulin. As in insulin, it also has three disulphide bonds but it has only a single chain of 70 amino acids rather than 51 of insulin. It is also called somatomedin C. Its major role is in childhood growth and has anabolic effects even in adults. Its production is stimulated by growth hormone, and therefore, serves as important marker for growth hormone bioactivity. Its concentration is reduced in starvation, malnutrition, growth hormone insensitivity (growth hormone receptor mutation) The IGF-1 in the circulation is bound to IGF-1 binding proteins. The IGFBP-3 binds about 80% of the hormone in a ratio of 1:1.

Receptors

Insulin-like growth factor-1 binds to IGF-1 receptor which is tyrosine kinase. It can thus phosphorylate other proteins. It can also bind to insulin receptor. Structure of IGF receptor is similar to insulin receptor. It is formed of two α-subunits and two β-subunits.

α-subunits are linked with each other by a single disulphide bond whereas α-subunits are linked to β-subunits by two disulphide bonds. The α-subunits are extracellular while the β-subunits span the membrane and their cytoplasmic domains are responsible for signal transduction. On ligand, binding receptors are autophosphorylated and trigger signal transduction.

Function

Its function is just like insulin. The IGF-1 stimulates systemic body growth and has growth promoting effects on almost every cell in the body such as muscle, cartilage, bone, liver, kidney, nerves, skin, hematopoietic cell, and lung. Deficiency of either growth hormone or IGF-1 results in short stature. Humans deficient in IGF-1—Larson Dwarfs are treated with recombinant IGF-1. The IGF-1 may have possible role in protecting vasculature against oxidative stress.

Insulin-like growth factor-1 levels are used as surrogate marker for excessive growth hormone in patients with growth hormone secreting pituitary tumors (acromegaly). Following surgical/medical therapy, IGF-1 can be used to monitor response; remission/progression.

INSULIN-LIKE GROWTH FACTOR 2

It is closely related to IGF-1. It binds to a host of insulin-related receptors. Signaling mostly occurs via IGF-1 receptors, but when circulating levels are high, it can engage insulin receptor isoform A. Tumors of mesenchymal and epithelial origin produce abundant IGF-2 resulting in fasting hypoglycemia similar to that seen in insulin producing tumors except that both insulin and growth hormone levels are suppressed. Surgical correction offers relief from hypoglycemia.

There have been speculations about liver producing factors that are important in glucoregulation. Exclusive role of integrity of insulin receptor in glucose homeostasis is being revisited.

CHAPTER 14

Hormones from Kidney

Kidney plays an important role in hormone production and degradation. It also happens to be an important site for hormone action (target sites). It is responsible for synthesis of two important hormones:
1. Erythropoietin
2. Calcitriol (1,25-dihydroxyvitamin D3): An active form of vitamin D essential for calcium homeostasis. This is accomplished through aegis of enzyme 1α - hydroxylase.

Additionally, kidney provides serine proteases-kallikreins that act on blood proteins to produce vasodilating peptide bradykinin. Kidney also secretes renin, a key enzyme in renin-angiotensin system. Renin is produced in the juxtaglomerular cells of the kidney. Kidney also produces many locally acting hormones (autocrine/paracrine regulators) such as prostaglandins (PGs), endothelin, and adrenomedullin. Most of these are important for blood pressure regulation. Kidney is also target for many important hormones: parathyroid hormone, aldosterone, angiotensin, and natriuretic peptides. Insulin is metabolized by kidneys and also excreted through kidneys. C-peptide is entirely metabolized/cleared by the kidneys.

ERYTHROPOIETIN

As the name indicates, this hormone is concerned with erythropoiesis (erythrocyte formation). It is produced by the interstitial fibroblasts in the kidney of adults. It is also produced by liver in the fetal and perinatal period. It is essential for red blood cell production. In its absence, erythropoiesis does not take place. It inhibits red cell apoptosis in bone marrow.

It is a single chain polypeptide glycoprotein hormone of 34 kDa. In addition to its function as erythropoietic molecule, it plays an important role in the brain's response to neural injury and wound healing.

Mechanism of Action

It binds to its receptor on the red cell progenitor surface and activates Janus kinase 2 (JAK-2) signaling cascade.

Synthesis and Regulation

Normal concentration of erythropoietin in circulation is about 10 mU/mL which can increase 1,000 fold in hypoxic conditions. Its levels are regulated by oxygen availability in blood via feedback mechanism. Recombinant hormone is available for clinical use.

RENIN AND KALLIKREIN

In addition to erythropoietin, kidney produces two enzymes which are important in the production of angiotensin and bradykinin. These two enzymes are renin and kallikrein. These play a role in regulation of blood pressure. Both cleave α2-globulins to produce their specific products—angiotensin and bradykinin. The latter is a vasodilator with natriuretic and diuretic activity.

RENIN ANGIOTENSIN SYSTEM

Angiotensin is an oligopeptide hormone that causes vasoconstriction and a subsequent increase in blood pressure. It is derived from angiotensinogen which is synthesized in the liver and is an α2-globulin. Human angiotensinogen is formed of 453 amino acids. It is converted to angiotensin by renin, an enzyme synthesized in the kidney. Angiotensinogen is first converted to angiotensin I which is a decapeptide (Fig. 14.1). Renin cleaves peptide bond between leucine and valine of angiotensinogen to form angiotensin I. Angiotensin converting enzyme further removes 2 C-terminal amino acids to form angiotensin II. Angiotensin II is metabolized to form angiotensin III and IV, respectively by sequential removal of aspartate (Asp) and arginine (Arg) from N-terminus of angiotensin II.

Functions of Angiotensins

Angiotensins III and IV have lesser activity. Angiotensin I has no biological activity. In addition to its vasoconstrictive role, angiotensin II also produces aldosterone from adrenal cortex which increases sodium reabsorption from proximal

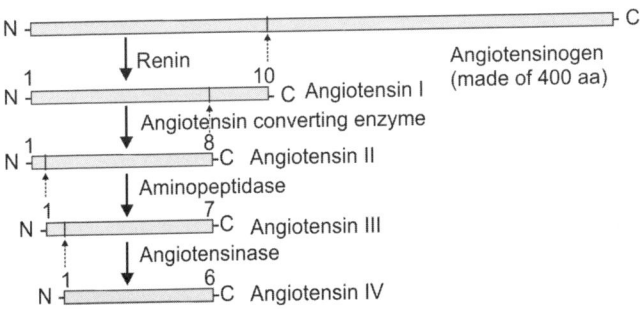

FIG. 14.1: Biosynthesis of angiotensins (dotted arrows show site of cleavage)

tubules of kidney. Angiotensin III is equally active in this regard. Angiotensin II also causes adhesion and aggregation of platelets.

Angiotensin Receptors

Angiotensin receptors are G-protein coupled receptors. These are of two types, AT1 and AT2. The AT1 is the major receptor and its G-protein α-subunit is G_q type which activates phospholipase C resulting into an increase in cytosolic calcium which in turn stimulates protein kinase C. Activated receptor also inhibits adenylate cyclase. All the functions of angiotensin II, such as vasoconstriction, aldosterone production, decreased renal blood flow, renal tubular Na^+ reabsorption, and renal renin inhibition, are mediated through AT1 receptor.

15
CHAPTER

Hormones from Heart

Heart is an important site for synthesis of peptides responsible for strong natriuresis (excretion of sodium), and thus, decongesting lungs and general circulation. In 1981, de Bold and his colleagues from Canada established that atrial muscle was the site of production for the hormone that came to be known as atrial natriuretic factor (ANF) or atrial natriuretic peptide (ANP). This peptide was isolated, purified, and sequenced from rat atrial extracts in 1983. In the following years, it was isolated from the human atria as well. This helped establish heart as an endocrine organ. Subsequently, related peptides, such as the brain natriuretic peptide (BNP) and C-type natriuretic peptide (CNP), were described. Other peptides, such as calcitonin gene-related peptide (CGRP), and endothelin-1 (ET-1), were found to be expressed in heart as well. These hormones, unlike ANP, are primarily serving autocrine/paracrine function.

Heart is an important target for thyroid hormone, and other hormones that are less characterized in terms of heart being the direct target.

ATRIAL NATRIURETIC PEPTIDE

Atrial natriuretic peptide as the name suggests is a peptide hormone secreted by atria of the heart and, regulates body sodium (natrium) level. It is also called atrial natriuretic factor or atriopeptin. It is a 28 amino acid peptide with a 17 amino acid ring in the middle formed by a disulphide bond between cysteine 7 and 23. Atrial natriuretic peptide is synthesized as a preprohormone of 151 amino acids which has a 25 amino acid signal peptide. Pro-atrial natriuretic peptide (ProANP) is converted to ANP by an enzyme named corin, a membrane serine protease. Atrial natriuretic peptide is also synthesized in ventricles, brain, suprarenal glands, and renal glands.

Lately, it has been shown that within the ANP prohormone, there are four hormones: long-acting natriuretic peptide, renal dilator, kaliuretic peptide, and ANP. All the four have anticancer effects.

Brain natriuretic peptide, also called B-type natriuretic peptide or ventricular natriuretic peptide, is a 32 amino acid peptide with a ring structure identical to ANP. It is secreted by the ventricles of the heart. Its name BNP pertains to because it was first found in pig brain. In humans, it is produced mainly in the ventricles. It is synthesized as a 134 amino acid preprohormone and converted to BNP-like PreproANP to ANP. Recently, a diagnostic test has been developed which can be used for screening of heart failure.

Functions

Atrial natriuretic peptide and BNP hormones of the atria and ventricles, respectively, counterbalance the renin angiotesin system. Acutely, they decrease blood pressure by:
- Increasing renal sodium and water excretion
- Stimulating vascular dilation
- Inhibiting aldosterone and renin secretion from adrenal cortex and kidney, respectively.

Chronically, ANP inhibits the hypertrophy of cardiac myocytes. Brain natriuretic peptide inhibits pressure induced ventricular fibrosis. Atrial natriuretic peptide causes lipolysis in adipose tissue, releasing free fatty acids.

Mechanism of Action

Atrial natriuretic peptide binds to its single transmembrane receptor whose cytosolic domain has intrinsic guanyl cyclase activity. The receptor has an extracellular domain, a single transmembrane region, and a 37 amino acid cytoplasmic domain. Its activation on binding ANP leads to formation of cyclic guanosine monophosphate which activates a protein kinase G. Protein kinase G activates a signaling pathway which inhibits actin myosin complex resulting into dilation of the blood vessel.

AAA System (Inter-relationship amongst Angiotensin, Aldosterone, and Atrial Natriuretic Peptide)

In response to increased osmolarity of the blood, juxtaglomerular cells release an enzyme, namely, renin. The latter acts on the protein angiotensinogen (produced by liver) and convert it into angiotensin I. Subsequently angiotensin I is converted to angiotensin II that causes release of aldosterone from the adrenal cortex. Aldosterone causes the reabsorption of sodium ions from distal convoluted tubule of the nephrons. This causes reabsorption of water by osmosis restoring the normal osmolarity of the blood. This is called renin angiotensin aldosterone system (RAAS).

Atrial natriuretic peptide released from atria of heart in response to increased blood pressure acts opposite to RAAS. This inhibits the reasorption of water from nephrons of the kidney, thus restoring blood pressure.

ENDOTHELIAL HORMONES (ENDOTHELINS)

Endothelins are a family of peptides which comprises endothelins 1–3. Each endothelin is formed of 21 amino acid residues. These are secreted by vascular endothelial cells. Infact, these were discovered from cultured endothelial cells. Endothelin-1 is synthesized as a proendothelin of 39 amino acids and converted to 21 amino acid mature peptide hormone by endothelin converting enzyme found on the endothelial cell membrane. Endothelin-1 formation and release are stimulated by antidiuretic hormone, angiotensin II, thrombin, and reactive oxygen species, and inhibited by ANP, nitric oxide, and prostacyclins.

Function

Endothelins are most potent vasoconstrictors and cause hypertension.

Mechanism of Action

Endothelins bind to their receptors called ET_A and ET_B. Both are G-protein coupled receptors and their G-protein α-subunit is G_q. Receptors on activation result into release of second messenger inositol triphosphate which causes release of calcium ions from sarcoplasmic reticulum causing smooth muscle contraction.

SUGGESTED READING

1. Vesely DL. Journal of investigative Medicine. Published 10th December. 2015.

CHAPTER 16

Vitamin A

Vitamin A, like vitamin D has a dual role. It plays a role in vision as well as a hormone. Vitamin A is derived from β-carotene which is an isoprenoid or a terpenoid. It has three different forms as shown in the figure 16.1. Retinoic acid (which acts like a hormone) is derived by oxidation from retinol via retinal. It acts like hormone in control of cell growth during embryonic development and oncogenesis. Its actions are mediated by binding to its receptor called retinoic acid receptor (RAR). This is a nuclear receptor of 432 amino acid residues. It acts as a transcription factor. It is activated by both all-trans retinoic acid and 9-cis retinoic acid. There are three RAR receptors α, β, and γ. Retinoic acid receptor is present in nucleus as a heterodimer with retinoic acid X receptor (RXR) and in the absence of ligand, the heterodimer binds to hormone response element complexed with a corepressor protein. On ligand binding, RAR dissociates from corepressor and binds with coactivator protein which promotes transcription resulting into the synthesis of messenger ribonucleic acid and proteins which play role in control of cellular growth.

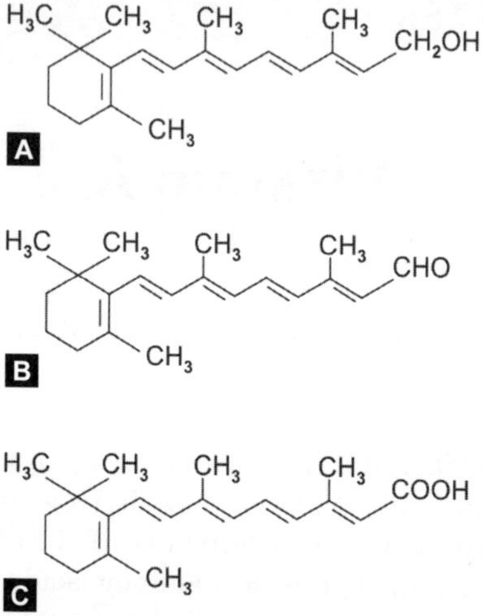

FIG. 16.1: Major forms of vitamin A. **A,** retinol; **B,** retinal; **C,** all-trans retinoic acid

CHAPTER 17

Prostaglandins

Prostaglandins are derived from arachidonic acid, which is a 20-carbon unsaturated fatty acid with four double bonds. It is released from diacylglycerol (DAG) by the action of enzyme phospholipase A2. In DAG, arachidonic acid is present at position 2. Arachidonic acid is acted upon by cyclooxygenase which produces prostaglandins. It is also acted upon by other enzymes which results into the production of prostacyclins, thromboxanes, and leukotrienes. All these together are called eicosanoids (having 20-carbon atoms).

The name prostaglandins were derived from the fact that these were first formed in prostate gland. Later on, it was realized that these are produced by seminal vesicles. All prostaglandins are derivatives of hypothetical 20-carbon prostanoic acid (Fig. 17.1). It has cyclopentane ring structure with two side chains (R1 and R2). R1 has carboxyl group and represents C1–C7 of prostanoic acid except in prostacyclins where R1 is C1–C5. R2 represents C13–C20 of prostanoic acid.

Prostaglandins differ due to nature of substituents and position of double bond on the cyclopentane ring. A subscript numeral denotes the number of double bonds in the two side chains and the subscript α denotes that the –OH group on C9 of ring and -COOH group are on the same side of the ring.

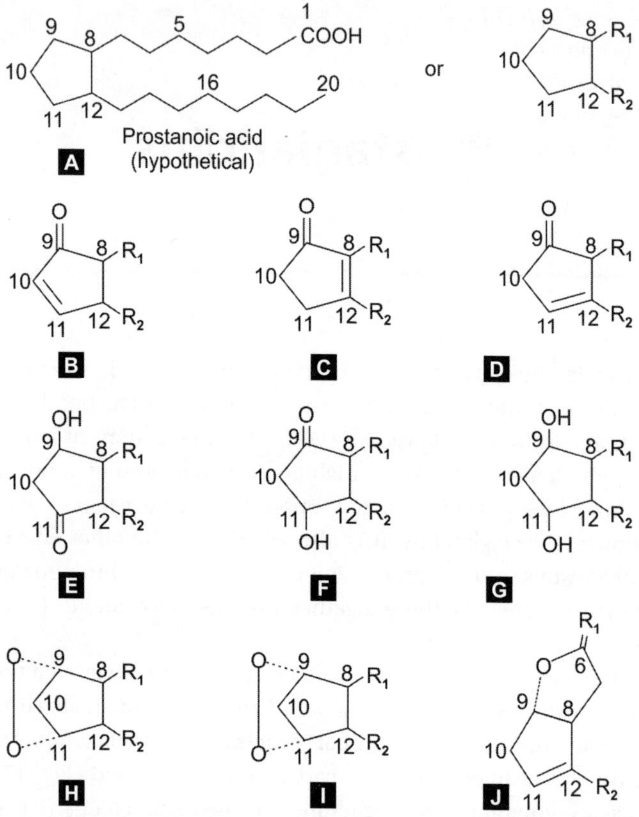

FIG. 17.1: Prostaglandins. **A,** prostanoic acid (hypothetical); **B,** prostaglandin A; **C,** prostaglandin B; **D,** prostaglandin C; **E,** prostaglandin D; **F,** prostaglandin E; **G,** prostaglandin F; **H,** prostaglandin G; **I,** prostaglandin H; **J,** prostacyclin

MECHANISM OF ACTION

Prostaglandins act either in an autocrine or paracrine manner locally. Their half-life is very short. Their receptors belong to subfamily of G-protein coupled receptors. These receptors have been termed DP1–2, EP1–4, FP, IP1–2 and TP corresponding to the receptor-ligand interaction, e.g., DP1–2 receptors bind prostaglandin D2. They are mediators of many physiological functions such as contraction and relaxation of smooth muscle, induce labor, regulate inflammation, calcium movement, hormone secretion, and cell growth. These are so important compounds that a Nobel Prize was awarded in 1982 for research on prostaglandins (see Nobel Prizes in endocrinology).

18
CHAPTER

Nitric Oxide

In 1992, Nobel prize was awarded for discovering the important biological function of nitric oxide (NO) in the fields of neuroscience, physiology, and immunology. It was proclaimed "molecule of the year" in 1992.

Nitric oxide is also known as nitrogen monoxide. It is a free radical and is produced by many cells of the body. In mammals, it is an important cellular signaling molecule. It is a powerful vasodilator. Its half-life in blood is only a few seconds.

It is also known as endothelium-derived relaxing factor. Endothelium (inner lining) of the blood vessels uses NO to signal the surrounding smooth muscle to relax, causing vasodilation and thus increasing blood flow. Nitric oxide acts in an autocrine as well as paracrine manner. It is produced from arginine by enzyme nitric oxide synthase (Fig. 18.1) as given below.

$$\text{L-arginine} + \text{NADPH} \rightarrow \text{NO} + \text{Citrulline}$$

MECHANISM OF ACTION

Nitric oxide after its formation in the endothelial cell diffuses into the surrounding smooth muscle where it activates enzyme guanylyl cyclase. The latter converts guanosine triphosphate to cyclic guanosine monophosphate (cGMP) which activates cGMP

Nitric Oxide

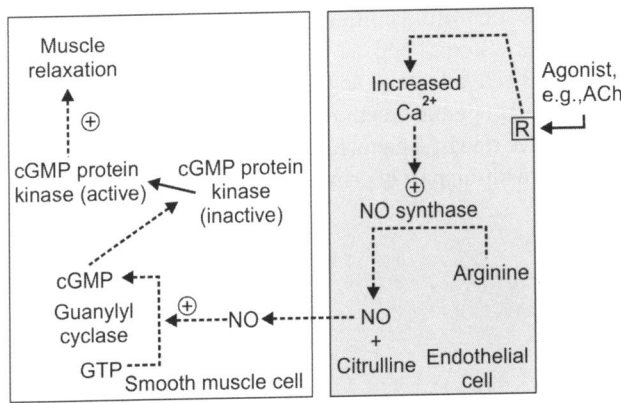

cGMP, cyclic guanosine monophosphate; GTP, guanosine triphosphate; NO, nitric oxide; R, receptor; ACh, acetylcholine.

FIG. 18.1: Formation and mechanism of action of nitric oxide

dependent protein kinase resulting in muscle relaxation. It binds to a soluble receptor guanyl cyclase (heterodimer made of one α-subunit and one β-subunit present in the cytoplasm). On activation, it increases intracellular levels of cGMP which then leads to vasodilation. Cyclic guanosine monophosphate activates protein kinase G which causes reuptake of calcium ions and opens calcium activated potassium channels. The fall in calcium levels ensures that the myosin light chain kinase can no longer phosphorylate the myosin molecule, thereby stopping the cross bridge cycle and leading to the relaxation of the smooth muscle.

PHYSIOLOGICAL FUNCTIONS OF NITRIC OXIDE

- Acts as an important vasodilator and thus helps in the regulation of blood pressure

- Acts as neurotransmitter in the brain and peripheral nervous system (PNS)
- Inhibits activation and aggregation of platelets
- Involved in penile erection
- Can have role in skeletal muscle relaxation
- Can constitute part of primitive immune system.

CHAPTER 19

Endocrine Tumors

INTRODUCTION

Endocrine tissue is as susceptible to neoplasia as nonendocrine tissue, with a difference that hormonal excesses (where the tumor is biologically active and producing hormones in excess) provide early signature of pathology, and hence, possible early diagnosis. Where the tumor is not active, its presence may be suggested by symptoms related to pressure on surrounding tissue which impacts the function of tissue/structures that are impinged upon. In many instances, endocrine tumors are detected incidentally while searching for pathology unrelated to the gland where tumor is detected (incidentaloma). Such discoveries may be lifesaving in that early treatment can change the course of potentially serious disease that might have gone unnoticed otherwise.

Endocrine tumors can present in following manner:
- Hormone oversecretion syndrome (depending on which hormone is oversecreted)
- Hormone hyposecretion by causing damage to surrounding tissues affecting their hormone production. Typically seen with pituitary tumors

---

This chapter has been exclusively contributed by Dr Romesh Khardori and Dr Ravneet Boparai

- Pressing on surrounding vital structures and affecting their function directly or affecting perfusion of surrounding tissue (particularly, in case of pituitary or suprasellar tumors that impinge on surrounding cranial nerves leading to cranial neuropathy).

Endocrine tumors may arise secondary to defects at target sites for hormone action. Therefore, a detailed history from the patient becomes very important. An example would be pituitary tumors arising in people with congenital adrenal hyperplasia which is primarily a steroid biosynthesis disorder.

Tumors may arise from any of the following sites:
- Pituitary: Adenoma (benign); carcinoma (malignant)
- Thyroid: Hyperplasia, follicular adenoma, follicular carcinoma, anaplastic carcinoma, medullary thyroid carcinoma
- Parathyroid: Hyperplasia, adenoma (benign), carcinoma
- Adrenal glands: Adenoma, hyperplasia, carcinoma, myelolipoma, pheochromocytoma
- Pancreas: Insulinoma, glucagonoma, gastrinoma, somatostatinomas, PPoma (pancreatic polypeptide producing).

PITUITARY TUMORS

Majority of pituitary tumors are benign adenomas. Pituitary carcinomas are very rare. A tumor less than 10 mm in size is called microadenoma while a tumor greater than 10 mm size is called macroadenoma. Both are capable of secreting hormones and clinical manifestation depends on the type of hormone produced [prolactin, growth hormone, adrenocorticotropic hormone (ACTH), thyroid stimulating hormone (TSH), and gonadotropin]. Macroadenomas can lead to pressure symptoms mostly involving the optic chiasm. Most common pituitary adenoma is prolactin secreting tumor (prolactinoma). It is easily identified by measuring prolactin level in blood. Typically, it affects young women who present with menstrual abnormalities, nipple discharge (milk-galactorrhea), and headaches. Medical treatment is often very effective.

Growth hormone secreting adenomas tend to be bigger when first diagnosed. Tumors occurring in childhood are associated with features of gigantism, while tumors appearing during adulthood are associated with classic features of acromegaly. Diagnosis is made by demonstrating tumor on imaging studies of sella and suprasellar lesion. Growth hormone and insulin-like growth factor 1 (IGF-1) levels are elevated. Gold standard for diagnosis is the demonstration of failure to suppress growth hormone level or paradoxical increase in growth hormone following administration of glucose load. Surgery is first-line treatment.

Adrenocorticotrophic hormone secreting adenoma results in excess blood levels of ACTH combined with elevated plasma cortisol levels. The clinical picture is typical of Cushing's syndrome (central obesity, moon facies, abdominal striae, hypertension, hirsutism and menstrual irregularity in females, and elevated blood glucose). When pituitary ACTH hypersecretion is the cause of Cushing's syndrome, it is called Cushing's disease. Surgical excision of tumor is the first line of treatment.

Thyrotropin hypersecreting adenomas lead to hyperthyroid state (hyperthyroidism) with inappropriately normal of mildly elevated blood TSH levels. These tumors are called TSHomas. Surgery is the most definitive first-line treatment.

Other pituitary hypersecreting disorders may result in elevation of gonadotropins [follicle stimulating hormone (FSH), luteinizing hormone].

A significant number of pituitary adenomas are non-secretory (nonfunctioning pituitary adenomas), and they come to attention often by virtue of neurovascular pressure symptoms arising from expanding tumor mass pressing on neighboring structures or rapid expansion of mass caused by hemorrhage within mass (apoplexy).

Pituitary tumors may be part of constellation of tumors in multiple endocrine glands [multiple endocrine neoplasia-1 (MEN-1)]. It is caused by inactivating mutation of *MEN-1* tumor suppressor gene located on chromosome 11q13 where germ line mutation has inactivated one allele, and the tumor occurs when second allele is silenced by a somatic mutation. The gene encodes menin which is important for deoxyribonucleic acid replication and transcription. The tumors arise from pituitary, parathyroid, pancreas, thymus, and adrenal glands (cortical). Pituitary tumor in MEN1 patients are present in 10–60% case, and may be the first clinical manifestation in about 15% cases. Prolactin secreting (60%) and growth hormone secreting (25%) tumors are the most frequent. The *MEN1* gene mutation can be found in 70–95% cases. About 90% cases have primary hyperparathyroidism.

There are other less common familial pituitary tumor syndromes—familial isolated pituitary adenoma; Carney complex; somatotropinoma/paraganglioma, X-linked acrogigantism, pituitary blastoma syndrome.

Familial isolated pituitary adenoma is identified by the presence of pituitary adenomas in two or more members of a family. In 20% of these families, a mutation is found on aryl-hydrocarbon receptor interacting protein (*AIP*) gene. In patients younger than 18 years, *AIP* mutations are found in 20% cases. The *AIP* mutation positive patients often tend to be males, have larger and invasive tumors, and 85% of these tumors are growth hormone or growth hormone/prolactin secreting tumors.

Carney complex, an autosomal dominant syndrome, is characterized by blue nevus, freckles, lentiginosis, spotty pigmentation, cardiac tumors (myxoma), acromegaly, thyroid carcinoma, pigmented nodular adrenocortical disease (PPNAD) with Cushing's syndrome. It is caused by an inactivating mutation in the regulatory subunit 1-α of the protein kinase A (PRKARIA). Cushing's syndrome due to PPNAD is the main endocrine manifestation (60%), followed by acromegaly.

THYROID GLAND

Tumors of thyroid gland include single (solitary) or multiple benign adenomas, as well as thyroid carcinoma [papillary, follicular, anaplastic, and medullary carcinoma thyroid (MCT)]. Often the patient is asymptomatic and without any overt circulating hormonal abnormalities. Thyroid cancer is often discovered incidentally when investigating patient with enlarged thyroid gland or evaluating patients with compression symptoms (change in quality of voice, difficulty with swallowing or breathing). Given widespread use of thyroid ultrasonography, most lesions can be biopsied and diagnosis made whether pathology is benign or malignant. Medullary thyroid carcinoma may be sporadic or part of genetic syndrome (MEN2) which represents a constellation of tumors of thyroid C-cells, parathyroid gland, and adrenal medullary tissue. This syndrome is a consequence of activating mutation of RET proto-oncogene located at 10q11.2. A combination of MCT, parathyroid hyperplasia, and pheochromocytoma is known as Sipple syndrome or MEN2A. Combination of MCT, pheochromocytoma, and ganglionenuromas is called MEN2B. Ganglioneuromas often precede MCT.

For most thyroid tumors, surgery is the best initial option. In thyroid cancer that has spread beyond confines of the thyroid gland, or exceeds a dimension of 7 cm, adjuvant radioactive iodine treatment is often recommended.

PARATHYROID GLAND

Often, parathyroid tumors are solitary and benign except when they are associated with MEN1 (less common with MEN2) where multiple glands are affected. Often, adenoma is associated with elevated level of circulated parathyroid hormone and calcium. This state is referred to as primary hyperparathyroidism. In a subgroup of benign parathyroid adenomas, *PRAD1* or *cyclin D1* gene have been implicated in tumor genesis. Retinoblastoma tumor suppressor gene (*RB*), another cell cycle regulator, has functional links to PRAD1. Abnormal RB protein expression is reported in a significant number of patients with cancer of parathyroid (parathyroid carcinoma).

Parathyroid glands may be enlarged in response to low systemic calcium levels seen in association with vitamin D deficiency (secondary hyperparathyroidism). Vitamin D repletion with restoration of calcium levels is often successful in treating secondary hyperparathyroidism. For primary hyperparathyroidism, surgery is the most definitive treatment. There are age-specific recommendations for surgery and chronic surveillance. Occasionally, ectopic secretion of parathyroid hormone may be the cause of parathyroid hormone driven hypercalcemia.

PANCREATIC TUMORS

Many of these tumors are benign. Clinical interest arises from symptoms associated with hypersecretion of pancreatic cell product [insulin hypersecretion (insulinoma)] leading to hypoglycemia. Diagnosis is confirmed by demonstration of elevated levels of fasting plasma insulin and C-peptide in conjunction with hypoglycemia. Excess production of glucagon, glucagonoma results in marked hyperglycemia and necrolytic cutaneous rash. Surgery is the treatment of choice. Other tumors of interest include gastrinoma, somatostatinomas, PPoma, and VIPomas (vasoactive intestinal peptide secreting). Unusually, pancreatic neuroendocrine tumors (PNETs) may participate in emergence of other syndromes such as Cushing's syndrome, carcinoid syndrome, and acromegaly.

Pancreatic neuroendocrine tumors have caught fancy of cell biologists and geneticists. Previously, PNETs were presumed arise from Langerhans cells. Now, the true genesis occurs in pluripotent stem cells of pancreatic acini/duct. The most important genetic alterations in PNET occur in *MEN-1* (multiple endocrine neoplasia-1), death-Domain associated protein/mental retardation syndrome X-linked genes (*DAXX/ATRX*), and the mammalian target of rapamycin (*mTOR*) pathway.

ADRENAL TUMORS

Those arising from adrenal cortex involve excessive secretion of aldosterone [primary hyperaldosteronism (Conn's syndrome)] cortisol (Cushing's syndrome). Tumor arising from adrenal medulla includes pheochromocytoma. Cortical tumors may be sporadic or part of MEN1 complex whereas pheochromocytoma may be a manifestation of MEN2 complex. Typically, these tumors present with accelerating or resistant hypertension in association with hypokalemia. Like most hypersecreting endocrine tumors (except prolactinoma), surgery is most favored initial treatment of choice.

MISCELLANEOUS

Tumors can arise in ovaries and testis as well that may be hypersecreting, but these are very uncommon. Hormonal hypersecretion may be secondary to ectopic secretion of peptides by nonendocrine neoplastic tissue such as seen in small cell carcinoma of lung and the carcinoid. Cases have been reported where a pituitary adenoma secreting gonadotropin (FSH) caused hypersecretion of gonadal steroids (ovarian as well as testicular).

ECTOPIC PEPTIDE HORMONE PRODUCTION

Peptide hormones may be secreted from some tumors, resulting in clinical presentation almost identical to that seen with oversecretion of hormone from its parent site. These are referred to as paraneoplastic syndromes. Such ectopic hormone production is surprisingly common and often seen in small cell lung cancers. These tumors may produce hormones like ACTH, arginine-vasopressin, parathyroid hormone-related protein, calcitonin, and β-human chorionic gonadotropin (β-hCG). Alternatively, releasing factors such as corticotropin releasing factor and growth hormone releasing hormone may be synthesized. When produced in excess, β-hCG may induce hypermetabolic state from secondary thyrotoxicosis because of its structural similarity with thyrotropin (TSH).

SUGGESTED READINGS

1. Clinical Endocrinology; Saffron Whitehead and John Miell. Scion Publishing Ltd. 2013.
2. Vassiliadi DA, Tsagarakis S. Endocrine Incidentalomas–Challenges imposed by incidentally discovered lesion. Nat Rev Endocrinol. 2011;7:668-80.
3. Leidig-Bruckner G. Endokrine Tumoren (article in German): Radiologe. 2014;54:966-74.
4. Syro LV, Rotondo F Ramirez A, Di Ieva A, Sav MA, Restrepo LM, et al. Progress in the diagnosis and classification of pituitary adenomas. Front Endocrinol (Lausanne). 2015;6:97.
5. Viúdez A, De Jesus-Acosta A, Carvalho FL, Vera R, Martín-Algarra S, Ramírez N. Pancreatic neuroendocrine tumors: Challenges in an underestimated disease. Critical Rev. Oncol Hematol. 2016;101:193-206.
6. Williams D. Inherited Susceptibility to Endocrine Neoplasia. In: Sheaves R, Jenkins PJ, Wass, JAH (Eds). Clinical Endocrine Oncology. New Jersey: Blackwell Science; 1997. pp. 30-7.

20
CHAPTER

Growth Factors

INTRODUCTION

Growth factors are being discussed in this text because these also act like hormones. They bind to their respective receptors and cause signal transduction. Mostly, they act either in paracrine or autocrine manner. Most of these growth factors are small proteins in nature and their major function is cell proliferation and differentiation in multicellular organisms. Following is the list of some important growth factors:

- Epidermal growth factor (EGF)
- Platelet-derived growth factor (PDGF)
- Nerve growth factor (NGF)
- Transforming growth factor-β (TGF-β)
- Fibroblast growth factor (FGF)
- Hepatocyte growth factor (HGF)
- Placental growth factor (PLGF)
- Vascular endothelial growth factor (VEGF)
- Thrombopoietin
- Insulin-like growth factor (IGF)-1 and IGF-2. Insulin itself is also a growth factor and causes cellular differentiation.

EPIDERMAL GROWTH FACTOR

It is a small soluble peptide growth factor of 53 amino acids with a molecular weight of 6,045 Da. It has three intermolecular disulphide bonds. It was first purified from mouse submandibular gland but later shown to be present in parotid gland also. It is also present in platelets and macrophages. It is produced by proteolytic cleavage between repeated EGF domains in the precursor protein. Precursor protein is anchored in the cell membrane spanning domain. Its function is to cause cell division. It binds to cells in the embryo, skin, and connective tissue in adults. Stanley Cohen and Rita Levi-Montalcini were given Nobel Prize in 1986 for discovering EGF.

Epidermal growth factor is the main founding member of EGF family. All the members have one or more repeats of conserved amino acid sequence (CX_7CX_4-$5CX_{10-13}CXCX_8GXRC$, where X represents any other amino acid). Some members include heparin binding EGF-like growth factor, TGF-α, neuregulin 1–4, amphiregulin, etc.

Mechanism of Action

Epidermal growth factor binds with high affinity with epidermal growth factor receptor (EGFR) situated on the cell surface. This causes dimerization and activation of intrinsic tyrosine kinase activity of EGFR. This activates Ras-Raf-MAPK pathway (Fig. 20.1) that results in variety of biochemical changes within a cell which includes increased protein synthesis and glycolysis, rise in intracellular calcium levels and increased expression of genes for EGFR. All these changes lead to increased deoxyribonucleic acid synthesis and cell proliferation.

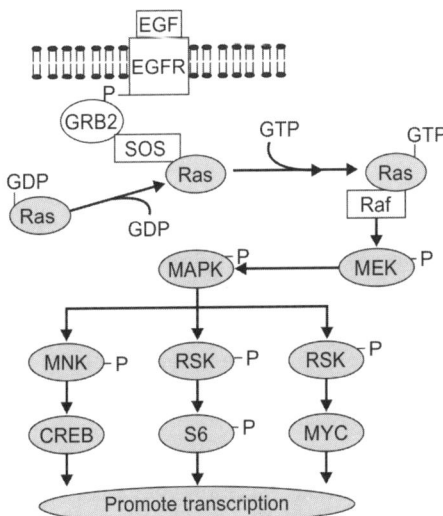

EGFR, epidermal growth factor receptor; EGF, epidermal growth factor; GRB2, growth factor receptor-bound protein 2; GTP, guanosine triphosphate; GDP, guanosine diphosphate; Ras, ribosomal protein S6 kinase; MAPK, mitogen-activated protein kinase; MAPK-interacting kinases.

FIG. 20.1: Mechanism of action of epidermal growth factor

PLATELET-DERIVED GROWTH FACTOR

There are at least four PDGFs, namely, PDGFA, PDGFB, PDGFC, and PDGFD. These are encoded by separate genes and PDGFA and PDGFB can form homo or heterodimers—AA, BB, and AB. These are produced by platelets, vascular cells, monocytes, macrophages, fibroblasts, and skin epithelial cells. They act in a paracrine manner and cause connective tissue cell proliferation and chemotaxis. Platelet-derived growth factors also induce replication and collagen synthesis by osteoblasts. Their receptors are tyrosine kinases. Ligand binding leads to receptor dimerization and activated receptor causes signal transduction by activating many pathways.

Mechanism of Action

Upon activation by PDGF, its receptor dimerizes to initiate signal transduction. Mechanism of action of PDGF is shown in figure 20.2. Receptor dimerization is followed by autophosphorylation and formation of high affinity sites of binding of signaling molecules such as growth factor receptor-bound protein 2. The latter associates with SOS to

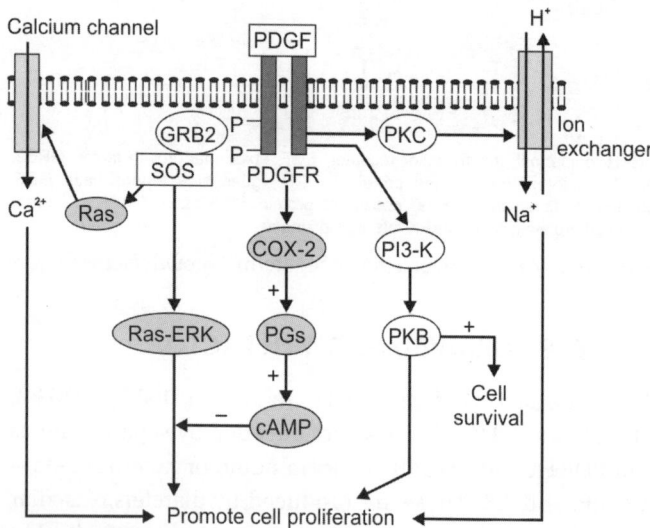

PI3-K, phosphatidylinositol 3-kinase; PKC, protein kinase C; COX, cyclo-oxygenase; PKB, protein kinase B; PG, prostaglandins; GRB2, growth factor receptor-bound protein 2.

FIG. 20.2: Mechanism of action of platelet-derived growth factor in hepatic cell

activate downstream signaling pathways which include Ras-ERK pathway, PI 3-K pathway, calcium/calmodulin, and protein kinase C dependent Na$^+$/Ca^{2+} exchanger.

Biological Functions

- During early development, PDGFs are mitogenic promoting the proliferation of undifferentiated mesenchyme cells
- During late development stages, PDGFs help in tissue remodeling and cellular differentiation
- Platelet-derived growth factor is required for cell division of fibroblasts in connective tissue which is helpful in wound healing process.

NERVE GROWTH FACTOR

Nerve growth factor was the first growth factor discovered from mouse sarcoma tumor and purified from submaxillary gland of mouse. For the discovery of growth factors, Stanley Cohen and Rita Levi-Montalcini were awarded Nobel Prize in 1986. It is a homodimer of two 118 residue polypeptides. It is a member of NGF family which also includes brain-derived neutrophic factor (BDNF) and neurotrophins (NT) 3, 4, and 5. Their receptors are tyrosine kinases (Trks); TrkA, TrkB and TrkC bind NGF, BDNF and NT3, respectively. On binding the ligand, the receptor provides a survival signal for neurons. It is said that without NGF, neurons commit suicide in cell culture. Thus, NGFs play an important role in differentiation and survival of neurons. Another receptor, p75 NTR, also binds these growth factors but with lower affinity. Both, TrkA and TrkB, can complex with p75 NTR and form a high affinity functional receptor. The TrkB expression is widespread throughout central nervous system.

Transforming Growth Factor-β

Transforming growth factor-β exists in an at least five isoforms (TGF-β 1–5). Each TGF-β is synthesized as a larger precursor that contains a prodomain. This prodomain is cleaved but remains noncovalently associated with the mature domain after TGF-β is secreted. Secreted TGF-β is stored in extracellular matrix as a latent inactive complex containing the cleaved TGF-β precursor and covalently bound TGF-β binding protein called latent TGF-β binding protein (LTBP). Activation of mature dimeric TGF-β requires dissociation of LTBP. It is achieved by binding of LTBP by the matrix protein thrombospondin or by certain cell surface integrins which cause conformational change in LTBP and LTBP is removed. Certain matrix and metalloproteinases can digest LTBP resulting in activation of mature TGF-β. The peptide structures of TGF-β isoforms are highly similar. The mature TGF-β1 is a dimer of two chains having 112–114 amino acids. The major function of TGF-β is to inhibit cell proliferation. It induces apoptosis of numerous cell types. It stops cell cycle at G1 stage to stop cell proliferation. The TGF-β acts through SMAD pathway by binding to its receptors (See SMADS). Loss of TGF-β receptors or certain intracellular proteins of the signaling pathway releases cells from growth inhibition and results into tumor formation.

FIBROBLAST GROWTH FACTOR

At least 21 are known including acidic, basic, and keratinocyte growth factor (FGF-7). They induce cell growth, differentiation, and migration. These bind to heparin or heparin sulfate chains of proteoglycan and this complex binds cell surface receptors on target cells. This binding of FGF to proteoglycans protects it from its degradation. The FGF receptors are tyrosine kinases and are of four types (FGFR1-4). Each receptor binds a unique set of FGFs. The FGF receptors have an extracellular N terminal domain, a transmembrane domain, and an intracellular immunoglobulin like domains (D1-D3). Only D2 and D3 domains bind FGF. Activation of FGF receptors leads to signaling via multiple pathways including phospholipase C-γ. The FGFs play a role in the survival of neural cells, stimulate proliferation of fibroblasts, endothelial cells, and smooth muscle cells.

HEPATOCYTE GROWTH FACTOR

It is produced by embryonic connective tissue cells (mesenchyme) in the limb buds and helps in migration of myoblasts to limb buds. It is also called scatter factor (SF). Production of HGF is induced by FGF. It is a disulphide linked heterodimeric molecule. It acts in an endocrine or paracrine manner. Its receptor is expressed on epithelial cells and is a tyrosine kinase. This receptor is called MET. On ligand binding, MET activation leads to embryonic growth and development, differentiation, wound healing, and angiogenesis. The MET receptors are also expressed in bone cells. In osteoclasts, HGF increases Ca^{2+} and replication. It stimulates osteoclasts to enter cell cycle.

PLACENTAL GROWTH FACTOR

It is a member of VEGF family. It occurs at least in three forms (PLGF 1-3). PLGF-2 binds to heparin with high affinity. The PLGF 1 or 3 do not bind heparin. It is a homodimeric protein of 46-50 KDa. Two monomers are linked by disulphide bonds. Its main source during pregnancy is the placental trophoblast. It is also expressed in villous trophoblast. Its main functions are angiogenesis and vasculogenesis during embryogenesis. Its expression in human atherosclerotic lesions is associated with plaque inflammation.

VASCULAR ENDOTHELIAL GROWTH FACTOR

It is also a protein growth factor. It is a glycoprotein. It is disulphide linked homodimer. At least five different forms are known (VEGF A-E). Vascular endothelial growth factor production can be induced in cells that are not receiving enough oxygen. A cell deficient in oxygen produces a transcription factor hypoxia inducible factor (HIF) which stimulates the release of VEGF. Their major functions are vasculogenesis and angiogenesis, endothelial growth promoting cell migration and inhibiting apoptosis.

Overproduction of VEGF causes retinopathy. The VEGF act by binding to their receptors which are tyrosine kinases. These receptors are of three types—VEGFR 1-3. These receptors have an extracellular portion consisting of seven immunoglobulin like domains, a single transmembrane domain and an intracellular domain having tyrosine kinase activity. On ligand binding, receptors dimerize and become active through transphosphorylation. The most important VEGR receptor is VEGFR2. It mediates all the functions of VEGF.

THROMBOPOIETIN

Thrombopoietin is a protein produced mainly by liver and in a little less quantity by kidney. It is also called megakaryocyte growth and development factor. Its major function is to control platelet production. Thrombopoietin levels increase within 24 hours after the onset of thrombocytopenia (decreased level of platelets). It is synthesized as a precursor protein of 353 amino acids of which first 21 N-terminal amino acids act as a signal peptide. After removal of signal peptide, the remaining protein is glycosylated and has a molecular weight of 60–70 kDa. The first 53 amino acids of mature protein are required for biological activity. Thrombopoietin acts by binding to two members of Janus kinase (JAK) tyrosine kinase family JAK2 and TYK2 activating STAT proteins which in the nuclei act as transcription factors (see JAK-STAT pathway).

APPENDIX

HORMONE LEVELS

Hormone	Males	Females
Anti-Müllerian hormone (ng/mL)	–	0.0–6.8
Cortisol µg/dL	8 AM: 5–25 4 PM: 3–12	8 AM: 5–25 4 PM: 3–12
Dehydroepiandrosterone sulfate (µg/dL)	80–560	1–430
Estradiol (pg/mL)	10–45	10–257.8
Free testosterone (pg/mL)	8.9–42.5	0.02–3.09
Follicle stimulating hormone (mIU/mL)	1.4–18.1	1.5–116.3
Growth hormone (ng/mL)	0.06–5.0	0.06–5.0
β-human chorionic gonadotropin (mIU/mL)	<10	<10
17-hydroxyprogesterone (ng/mL)	0.6–3.34	0.11–5.0
Insulin levels fasting Postprandial (µIU/mL)	2–25 22–75	2–25 22–75
Luteinizing hormone (mIU/mL)	1.5–9.3	0.5–76.3
Progesterone (ng/mL)	0.28–1.22	0.15–25.56
Prolactin (ng/mL)	2.1–17.7	2.8–29.2
Parathyroid hormone (pg/mL)	15–65	15–65
Total testosterone (ng/mL)	2.41–8.27	0.14–0.76
Total triiodothyronine (ng/mL)	0.6–1.8	0.6–1.8
Total thyroxine (µg/dL)	5.0–12.45	5.0–12.45
Thyroid stimulating hormone (µU/mL)	0.35–5.0	0.35–5.0

Index

Page numbers followed by *f* refer to figure and *t* refer to table.

A

Acetylcholine 8, 147
  receptor 24, 31
Activin 110
Addison's disease 68
Adiponectin 120
  functions 121
  receptors 121
Adipose tissue 5, 65
  hormones 117
Adrenal
  cortex 62, 135
    pathophysiology of 68
  gland 62, 152
  insufficiency, secondary 69
  medulla 4, 71, 73*f*
    pathophysiology of 74
  tumors 155
Adrenocorticoids, synthesis of 64*f*
Adrenocorticosteroids
  biochemical functions 65
  biosynthesis of 63
Adrenocorticotropic hormone 31, 40-42, 150, 151
Aldosterone 139
Aldosteronism 70
Amylin 99
Androgen
  biochemical functions 105
  biosynthesis 104
  synthesis of 65
Angiotensin 134, 139
  biosynthesis of 135*f*
  converting enzyme 135
  functions of 135
  receptors 136

Angiotensinogen 135
Antidiuretic hormone 44, 45
  biochemical functions 45
Anti-Müllerian hormone 111
Atrial natriuretic
  factor 137
  peptide 137-139
    functions 138
Autoimmune
  destruction of β cells 100
  disease 31, 59
  hypoparathyrodism 80

B

Bacterial endotoxin 29
Bombesin 129
Bordetella pertussis 25
Bradykinin 134
Brain-derived neurotrophic factor 161

C

Calcitonin 60, 85
  biochemical functions 85
  gene-related peptide 137
Calcitriol 81
  biochemical functions 83
  biosynthesis of 82, 83*f*
  synthesis, regulation of 82
Calcium 77
  activated potassium channels 147
  homeostasis 133
  ions, reuptake of 147
  levels 154, 155
  metabolism 60

Calmodulin 27
Carbohydrate, metabolism of 91
Carboxypeptidase-like enzyme 89*f*
Carcinoid syndrome 154
Cardiac tumors 152
Catecholamines
   biochemical functions 74
   biosynthesis of 71
   synthesis of 73*f*
Central nervous system 123
Chemiluminescent microparicle immunoassay 17
Cholecalciferol 82
Cholecystokinin 126
Cholera toxin 29
Circadian rhythms 123
Conn's syndrome 70, 155
Cranial neuropathy 150
Cushing's disease 47
Cushing's syndrome 69, 151, 153, 154, 155
Cyclic adenosine monophosphate 26
Cyclic guanosine monophosphate 26, 147
Cyclo-oxygenase 160

D

Dehydroepiandrosterone 105
Deoxyribonucleic acid 7, 107
Diabetes 99, 101
   complications 101
   gestational 101
   insipidus 48
   mellitus 99
      type 1 100
      type 2 97, 99
Diacylglycerol 26, 27, 143
Diiodothyronine 53

E

Ectopic hormone production 35, 156

Eicosanoids 143
Endocrine
   glands 3, 3*t*, 5, 87
   neoplasia-1, multiple 152
   pancreatic disorders 99
   tissue 149
   tumors 149
Endocrinology 1
Endothelial hormones 140
Endothelins 140
Enkephalins 42
Enzyme coupled receptors 19
Enzyme-linked immunosorbent assay 16
Epidermal growth factor 158, 159, 159*f*
   receptor 159
Epididymal fat 14
Epinephrine 72, 90
Erythropoiesis 134
Erythropoietin 134
Escherichia coli 25
Estrogen 109
   biochemical functions 108
   biosynthesis 107, 108*f*
Exophthalmia 2

F

Familial
   glucocorticoid deficiency 31
   hyperaldosteronism 70
   pituitary tumor syndromes 152
      isolated pituitary adenoma 152
Fibroblast growth factor 162

G

Galactorrhea 151
Gastric inhibitory peptide 128
Gastrin 126
   biochemical functions 126
Gastrinoma 127, 154

Gastrointestinal
  tract 5, 125
    hormone 11, 90, 98, 129
Genetic defects 30, 31
Ghrelin 129
  functions of 129
Glucagon 5t, 10, 96
  functions of 97
Glucagon-like peptide 127, 128
Glucocorticoids
  cellular effects of 66
  functions of 65
  related disorders 68
  synthesis of 63
Glucose transporters 96
Glutamic acid 31
Glycosylated hemoglobin 102
Glycogen phosphorylase
    kinase 27
Glycoprotein hormones 6, 43
Glycosuria 100
Goiter 2, 57, 58
Gonadotroph adenoma 47
Gonadotropin 43
Gonadotropin-releasing
    hormone 34
Gonads 5, 104
G-protein 24
  coupled receptors 19, 20, 20f
Growth
  factor 157
    receptor-bound protein 2, 159
  hormone 30, 38, 132, 151
    biochemical functions 38
    prolactin group 38
Guanine nucleotide binding
    proteins 24
Guanosine
  diphosphate 159
  triphosphate 147, 159
Guanyl cyclase receptors 22

H

Hashimoto's thyroiditis 59
Heat shock protein 22
Hepatic cell 160f
Hepatocyte growth factor 163
Heterocrine gland 87
Hinge region 23
Hormone 1, 3, 77, 113t, 123, 137
  adipocyte-derived 122
  affinity 9
  assays 13
  autocrine 1
  binding domain 23
  chemical nature of 5
  classification 7
  follicle stimulating 6, 43, 107
  from heart 137
  function, endothelial 140
  glycoprotein 6, 43
  groups of 7, 8, 8t
  incretin 127
  inhibitory 110
  juxtacrine 1
  levels
    negative feedback control of 11
    positive feedback control of 13
  luteinizing 6, 31, 104
  luteotropic 40
  mammotropin 40
  melanocyte stimulating 42
  oversecretion syndrome 149
  paracrine 1
  peptide 6, 156
  polypeptide 6
  receptors 19
  replacement 49
  response element 107
Human
  chorionic gonadotropin 6, 113
  glucocorticoid receptor 66

Hyperparathyroidism 81
Hyperthyroidism 58
Hypervitaminosis D 84
Hypoglycemia 102
Hypogonadism
  primary 113
  secondary 114
Hypothalamic hormones 35
Hypothalamic-pituitary-adrenal axis 118
Hypothalamus 3, 33
Hypothyroidism 58
Hypoxia inducible factor 164

I

Incidentaloma 149
Inhibin 110
  receptors 110
Inositol triphosphate 26
Insulin 10, 30, 87, 89f
  action, mechanism of 92
  antibodies 31
  biochemical functions 91
  biosynthesis 88
  degradation 91
  hypersecretion 154
  in vitro assay of 14
  in vivo assay of 14
  receptor 21, 93f
    activated 94
    substrate 95
  release
    factors inhibiting 90
    factors promoting 89
    first phase of 90
  resistance 103
  secretion 89
  sensitivity 103
  signal transduction for 94f
  structure 88
Insulin-like growth factor 131, 132, 157

Intracellular receptor 20
  function 31
Iodide ion 52
Islet amyloid polypeptide 99
Islet of Langerhans 87

K

Kallikrein 134
Kallmann syndrome 115
Klinefelter's syndrome 114

L

Lambert-Eaton myasthenic syndrome 31
Laron dwarfism 30
Leprechaunism 30
Leptin 117
  functions of 118
  receptors 118
Leydig cells 104
Lipid metabolism 92
Lipotropin 42

M

Megakaryocyte growth factor 164
Melatonin receptors, subtypes of 123
Menstrual cycle 112, 113t
Mineralocorticoids
  associated disorders 70
  cellular effects of 68
  functions of 66
  synthesis of 63
Monoiodothyronine 52, 53
Motilin 128
Müllerian inhibiting factor 111
Myxoma 152

N

Natriuretic peptide
  B-type 138
  C-type 137

Index

Nerve growth factor 161
Nicotinamide adenine
dinucleotide phosphate 53
Nitric oxide 146, 147, 147f
  function of 146
  physiological functions of 147
Nonendocrine tissue 149

O

Organic acids 77
Oxidized iodide 52
Oxytocin 45
  biochemical functions 44
  structure of 44

P

Pancreas 4, 69, 87
Pancreatic
  neuroendocrine tumors 154, 155
  polypeptide 98
  tumors 154
Paragangliomas 75
Parathyroid gland 76, 153
  pairs of 78
  pathophysiology of 80
Parathyroid hormone 76, 78, 79, 81
  biochemical functions 79
  biosynthesis of 78
  formation of 78f
Peripheral nervous system 148
Phosphate 77
Phosphatidylinositol
3-kinase 160
Pineal gland 3, 123
Pinealocytes 123
Pituitary
  adenomas 151
  gland 37, 48
    anterior 4, 37
    intermediate 4
    pathophysiology of 46
    posterior 4, 44
  tumor 150, 152
Placenta 5
Placental growth factor 163
Plasma
  calcium 76
  membrane receptor 19
    interaction 30
Platelet-derived growth
factor 159, 160f
Platelets, decreased level of 165
Prediabetes 100
Preprohormones 10
Preproparathormone 78f
Progesterone 105
  biochemical functions 109
  biosynthesis 109
Proinsulin 89f
  structure of 89f
Prolactin 40, 150
  biochemical functions 40
Prolactinoma 150
Pro-opiomelanocortin
  gene products 42f
  peptide family 41
  products 41
Prostacyclin 144f
Prostaglandins 143, 144f
Protein kinase 160
  A 27, 97
  mitogen-activated 159
Pseudohypoparathyroidism 80

R

Radioimmunoassay 15
  standard curve 15f
Rat hemidiaphragm assay 14
Receptor tyrosine kinases 21
Renal rickets 84

Renin 134
  angiotensin
    aldosterone system 139
    system 135
Reproductive system, pathophysiology of 113
Retinal 142f
Retinoblastoma tumor 154
Retinoic acid
  all-trans 142f
  receptor 141
Retinol 142f
Ribosomal protein S6 kinase 159

S

Sleep cycles 123
Somatostatin 97
Steroid 22
  hormone 23
    receptor 23f
Sulfonylureas 101
Supraoptic nucleus 34
Suprarenal glands 62
Sympathetic nervous system 119

T

Tachyphylaxis 86
Testosterone 106
  synthesis 106f
Thrombopoietin 164
Thyroglobulin 52
Thyroid 4, 30
  function, evaluation of 56
  gland 50, 153
    pathophysiology of 57
  hormone 22, 55, 119
    biochemical functions of 54
    biosynthesis of 51, 53f
    metabolism of 54
    structure of 51
  medullary carcinoma 153
  stimulating hormone 6, 43, 150
    levels 57
Thyrotoxicosis 58
Thyrotropin-releasing hormone 34
Thyroxine 50
  binding globulin 52
  synthesis, regulation of 56
  transport of 52
Toxin-associated diseases 29
Transforming growth factor-β 162
Triiodothyronine 50
  synthesis, regulation of 56
  transport of 52
Trypsin-like enzyme 89f
Turner's syndrome 114

V

Vascular endothelial growth factor 164
Vasoactive intestinal peptide 127
Vasopressin 30, 45
  structure of 45
Ventral medial hypothalamus 119
Vibrio cholerae 25
Vitamin
  A 22, 141, 142f
  D 22, 81, 84, 141, 154
    deficiency 84
  D3 85

Z

Zollinger-Ellison syndrome 127
Zona
  fasciculata 62
  glomerulosa 62
  reticularis 62